WHY DO I HA
WHAT IS HAPPE
WHY DON'T DRUGS AND OTHER CONVENTIONAL
TREATMENTS MAKE ME FEEL BETTER?

Toxins, which are all around us, are at the root of many autoimmune diseases. They lurk in our clothing, our furniture, and in
the products we use every day. Our bodies make heroic efforts to
eliminate the toxins, but sometimes the burden is just too much.
Get the facts on:

- Bottled water: Toxins from the plastic bottles can leak into
  the water. Use a water filter instead.
- Plants: Did you know pollution-reducing plants, including
  mums and spider plants, can remove chemicals such as
  formaldehyde and benzene from the air?
- Toxins in your home: Carpets, furniture, plastics, foam rubber, upholstery, tiles, linoleum, paint, and varnishes emit
  hazardous chemicals into the air.
- Safe pest controls: Use boric acid and heat instead of toxic
  pesticides.
- Radiation: Protect yourself from the dangers of microwaves,
  computers, cell phones, televisions, power lines, heating
  pads, electric blankets, and more.

LEARN . . .
WHAT YOUR DOCTOR MAY *NOT* TELL YOU ABOUT

AUTOIMMUNE
DISORDERS

WHAT YOUR DOCTOR MAY *NOT* TELL YOU ABOUT

AUTOIMMUNE DISORDERS

The Revolutionary Drug-free Treatments for • Thyroid Disease • Lupus • MS • IBD • Chronic Fatigue • Rheumatoid Arthritis, and Other Diseases

---

STEPHEN B. EDELSON, M.D., and DEBORAH MITCHELL

A Lynn Sonberg Book

WARNER BOOKS

An AOL Time Warner Company

Warner Books, Inc., 1271 Avenue of the Americas, New York, NY 10020

Visit our Web site at www.twbookmark.com.

 An AOL Time Warner Company

Printed in the United States of America

First Printing: March 2003
10 9 8 7 6 5 4 3 2 1

Library of Congress Cataloging-in-Publication Data
Edelson, Stephen.
      What your doctor may not tell you about autoimmune disorders : the revolutionary drug-free treatments for thyroid disease, lupus, MS, IBD, chronic fatigue, rheumatoid arthritis, and other diseases / Stephen B. Edelson and Deborah Mitchell.
        p. cm.
      Includes index.
      ISBN 0-446-67924-0
      1. Autoimmune diseases—Alternative treatment. 2. Autoimmune diseases—Popular works. I. Mitchell, Deborah R. II. Title.

RC600 .E344 2003
616.97'806—dc21   2002068972

This book is dedicated to my wife, Carol, who has always been the major supporting structure in my endeavor to achieve the best in the work that I do, and to my children (Dana, Richard, Alex, Brad, and Joshua), who make me want to continue to "produce." Lastly, to my mother and deceased father, who were there from the beginning.

S.B.E.

This book is dedicated to my ever-patient husband, Tim Schaefer, and to Shiloh, my faithful feline companion during the writing of this manuscript, who succumbed to a fatal disease at the age of four and a half years as the book was completed.

D.M.

Acknowledgments

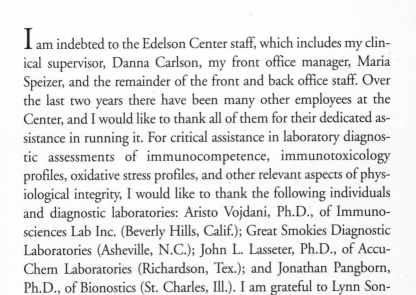

I am indebted to the Edelson Center staff, which includes my clinical supervisor, Danna Carlson, my front office manager, Maria Speizer, and the remainder of the front and back office staff. Over the last two years there have been many other employees at the Center, and I would like to thank all of them for their dedicated assistance in running it. For critical assistance in laboratory diagnostic assessments of immunocompetence, immunotoxicology profiles, oxidative stress profiles, and other relevant aspects of physiological integrity, I would like to thank the following individuals and diagnostic laboratories: Aristo Vojdani, Ph.D., of Immunosciences Lab Inc. (Beverly Hills, Calif.); Great Smokies Diagnostic Laboratories (Asheville, N.C.); John L. Lasseter, Ph.D., of Accu-Chem Laboratories (Richardson, Tex.); and Jonathan Pangborn, Ph.D., of Bionostics (St. Charles, Ill.). I am grateful to Lynn Sonberg for her guidance and for giving me the opportunity to write this book. Lastly, I wish to express my gratitude to all my patients, who have allowed me to learn so much in taking care of them. Without their help and courage I could not have unveiled the deeper levels of the biological disorders that underlie the disease.

Contents

Introduction   xi

PART I: UNDERSTANDING AUTOIMMUNITY

Chapter 1: What Is Autoimmunity?   3

Chapter 2: The Evaluation: How Do I Know If I Have an
           Autoimmune Disease?   27

PART II: COMMON AUTOIMMUNE DISEASES

Chapter 3: Autism   59

Chapter 4: Lupus   75

Chapter 5: Autoimmune Thyroid Disorders   98

Chapter 6: Rheumatoid Arthritis   117

Chapter 7: Crohn's Disease and Ulcerative Colitis   141

Chapter 8: Multiple Sclerosis   163

Chapter 9: Miscellaneous Autoimmune Disorders   185

Chapter 10: Chronic Fatigue and Immune Dysfunction
           Syndrome: A "Partial" Autoimmune Disease   207

PART III: TREATING AUTOIMMUNE DISEASES

Chapter 11: Biodetoxification: How to "Clean Your House"   235

Chapter 12: Nutritional Therapies   266

Chapter 13: Immunotherapy   297

Closing Comments   317

Glossary   320

Appendix   326

Worth Reading   337

Index   339

Introduction

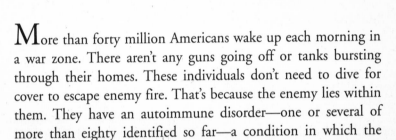

More than forty million Americans wake up each morning in a war zone. There aren't any guns going off or tanks bursting through their homes. These individuals don't need to dive for cover to escape enemy fire. That's because the enemy lies within them. They have an autoimmune disorder—one or several of more than eighty identified so far—a condition in which the body attacks its own cells and destroys them.

You know these disorders by names such as lupus, rheumatoid arthritis, scleroderma, multiple sclerosis, diabetes type 1, Crohn's disease, and thyroiditis, among others. These conditions largely affect women; in fact, about 75 percent of all autoimmune cases involve women, most often in their childbearing years. Among U.S. women, autoimmune disorders collectively are the fourth largest cause of disability, ranking behind cancer, heart disease, and mental illness. Clearly, autoimmune disease has a dramatic impact on lives.

You've probably picked up this book because you are one of the forty million. If you are like many of your fellow sufferers, you've been to two, three, even six or more doctors in search of answers to why you feel so poorly. When you recounted your story to a doctor—about your chronic fatigue, persistent muscle aches and pains, low-grade fever, dizziness, or how you generally feel lousy all or most of the time—you may have been told it was stress, or a part of aging, or depression. Then you may have been handed a prescription for a painkiller, a sleeping pill, or an antidepressant and sent on your way.

Maybe you were one of the "lucky" ones who found a doctor who ran a lot of tests and came up with a diagnosis for an autoimmune disease: for example, lupus, or thyroiditis, or rheumatoid arthritis. Then you felt validated; someone had named your disease. You went home with an armful of prescription bottles, but after months of taking pills and more pills, you still didn't feel good. Chances are you had side effects from some of the medications, and then you were given more drugs to treat those side effects. You felt caught in an endless cycle of pills, pain, and confusion.

Every day at the Edelson Center for Environmental and Preventive Medicine, I see people who were once caught in that endless cycle. They were caught there because the current approach to autoimmune diseases by the traditional medical community is based—like with most diseases—on treatment of the symptoms of the illness rather than removal of the cause. But, you ask, isn't it more logical to remove the cause than to just put a bandage on the symptoms, which doesn't make any attempt to heal the body?

Sure it is. But current medical school curriculum is based on a doctrine of medicine that dates back to the 1800s. That doctrine is founded on naming a disease and finding a medication or other treatment that will suppress it. This approach is not interested in identifying why a patient is ill, nor is it concerned with discovering ways to heal the body. Thus you and millions of others with autoimmune conditions are not being helped by conventional medicine, because doctors are not trying to remove the root cause of your disease: they only want to treat its symptoms. And that is only a temporary solution.

It's like a man who keeps cutting down the weeds in his lawn: if he really wants to get rid of the weeds, he needs to address the roots and either pull them out or permanently destroy them. But if he just keeps cutting off the tops of the weeds with his mower, they will keep coming back. Taking drugs to mask the symptoms of your autoimmune disease is just a temporary measure.

In 1982, I got tired of being that lawn mower. After years of practicing conventional medicine, I found myself faced with a large number of individuals who were suffering with all types of chronic illnesses, from rheumatoid arthritis to lupus, chronic fatigue syndromes, autoimmune hepatitis, autoimmune kidney disease, multiple sclerosis, type 1 diabetes, and others. And I came to the realization that the conventional approach was not working. I was not healing people; I was simply patching their wounds. There had to be a better way.

For years I scoured the research, looking for a way to help these patients. And what I began to piece together was a fascinating puzzle that pointed to a link between environmental toxins and the autoimmune process. Few people were doing the research, and the studies were in animals, but the evidence was convincing.

I then determined which components I believed were necessary to tackle this connection. Those components—applied immunology, applied toxicology, free-radical medicine, nutritional biochemistry, and environmental medicine—became the essence of what I call clinical molecular medicine, which I explain a bit more below. I began to use the diagnostic and treatment approaches discussed in this book on my patients, and I got results.

People were getting better and staying better. And hundreds of success stories later, it still works.

That's when I decided to share my success in a book.

At the Edelson Center, we heal bodies, and our record is fantastic. We have reversed or controlled nearly all the autoimmune diseases that have been presented to us, including Crohn's disease, chronic fatigue syndromes, multiple sclerosis, lupus, rheumatoid arthritis, chronic autoimmune renal disease, autoimmune thyroid gland disease, and others. Treatment is accomplished only when patients commit to the evaluation and the necessary course of treatment.

The word "environmental" in our name causes many people to pause. You may be wondering, what does the environment have to do with autoimmune disease?

I'm glad you asked. Because what makes the body turn upon itself is a combination of two factors: genetics (which is the hand we're dealt, so we have to learn to live and work with it); and environmental toxins.

Why do I believe environmental toxins are a major factor in autoimmune disorders? Because my years of experience have demonstrated to me that the body of every patient who has an autoimmune disorder is burdened with toxic chemicals and/or heavy metals. Because humans have seriously contaminated the three things we need to live: air, water, and food. And this contamination has taken place on a great scale and with increasing seriousness within the last hundred years—the same time period in which we have seen a dramatic rise in the prevalence and incidence of autoimmune disorders, as well as cancer and other deadly diseases.

Coincidence? I think not.

The promise of a better life through chemicals has, unfortunately, turned into a nightmare. There's arsenic in your drinking water, formaldehyde in the carpeting in your home and office and in your bedsheets, nickel in your peanut butter, toluene in your copy paper, and benzoic acid in your toothpaste. Environmental pollutants like mercury, lead, cadmium, tin, benzene, toluene, and formaldehyde have a wide spectrum of effects on the immune system, including autoimmunity, a condition that causes the cells in your body to attack themselves. Environmental pollutants can also cause a decrease in the system's ability to fight disease-causing organisms and tumors. The unfortunate truth is that there are more than 60,000 chemicals in the environment, with about 2,000 more being added every year.

That means they are in you, too. If you have the genetic makeup or susceptibility for autoimmunity, then those toxins can trigger your disease process. That's when you go looking for answers, relief, and healing, and don't find them. That's when you learn that the vast majority of doctors who treat autoimmune disorders simply attack the symptoms and, if they are lucky, hold the disease at bay. But a handful of us are addressing the root cause of these often debilitating diseases and getting lasting, healing results.

At the Edelson Center, for more than ten years, we have been providing an innovative treatment strategy that differs from that of conventional medical practitioners: we look at the cellular or molecular level of disease, an approach I call clinical molecular medicine.

Autoimmune disorders are very complex, so they require an intense, multilevel treatment approach. Clinical molecular medicine is a new, exciting field of medicine, and for nearly a decade I have been a part of it. It integrates four areas of study: environmental medicine (the study of the effects of the environment on human illness), applied immunology (the study of immune system functioning), toxicology (the study of free-radical biology and the toxins that may cause illness), and clinical nutritional biochemistry (the analysis of the chemical processes that may be inefficient in cell functioning). It takes such an integrated approach to deal with and heal from autoimmunity.

I believe that nearly all autoimmune diseases have their roots in toxicity: mercury, lead, and other heavy metals; poisonous chemicals like toluene; pesticides like DDT; and other environmental toxins like secondhand smoke and formaldehyde, all of which can help alter a person's immune system from a healthy, functional process into an autoimmune-type process.

Because nearly all autoimmune diseases have similar roots, my treatment approach has one overriding goal: to eliminate the toxins in the bodies of people with an autoimmune process. We focus on finding all the details concerning the basic mechanisms of a person's illness, and then develop molecular approaches to treat and prevent worsening disease or dysfunction. In essence, we find out why you are ill, not just the name of your condition. We treat the root cause, not just the symptoms.

In fact, I don't need to know which specific autoimmune disorder an individual has, because the label doesn't matter: it's the process at the cellular level that matters, and that is what I am treating. My treatment approach is safe to try regardless of the diagnosis. Exactly how I rid the body of toxins and return the body to health, however, differs for each individual and is based on his or her immune system, the toxins each person has been exposed to, the individual's unique detoxication system, and one's overall health.

For example, mercury is one of the most common metals in the environment that will cause the immune system to shift from operating on a healthy level to an unhealthy or autoimmune level, in which the body attacks itself. Mercury can be found in countless places: from auto exhaust to the amalgam fillings in your teeth, the water you drink, and the fish you may eat.

If you are exposed to high levels of mercury, or if your body cannot adequately get rid of the mercury it does take in, excessive amounts of molecules called free radicals (unstable molecules that can cause significant damage to the body) are formed, which lead to cell, tissue, and organ damage. Free radicals can be produced by various agents, including chemical toxins, heavy metals, and other environmental poisons. Symptoms of mercury toxicity (poisoning) include fatigue, depression, muscle and joint pain, dizziness, and headache, to name just a few. Do these sound familiar? People with autoimmune conditions such as lupus or rheumatoid arthritis will recognize them because they live with them. And they live with them because their immune systems have become dysfunctional.

My treatment approach is revolutionary because it is virtually 100 percent drug-free, is individually tailored for each patient, and consists of many different components, which are explained in detail in this book. One unique aspect of my diagnostic approach, for example, involves the use of an extensive proprietary Comprehensive Medical History Evaluation Questionnaire during which I ask individuals specific questions about their exposure to certain household, workplace, and other environmental toxins, a process not used by conventional physicians. This evaluation makes people take an in-depth look at their lives and gives me a treasure trove of information that is a critical part of my diagnostic process.

In the treatment category, one of the therapies I use is chelation therapy, which is a way to remove toxins such as mercury and lead from the body. Chelation therapy is practiced by more than a thousand medical doctors, osteopaths, and clinics across the country and can be highly effective in cleansing the body of poisons.

Another important and effective treatment for autoimmune diseases is antioxidant therapy, which is the use of over-the-counter substances such as vitamins C and E, glutathione, beta-carotene, lipoic acid, and many others, to help prevent cell damage in people who suffer with autoimmune disorders.

Hundreds and hundreds of people with lupus, rheumatoid arthritis, multiple sclerosis, diabetes type 1, and other auto-immune conditions have benefited from the treatments we use at the Center, and I share some of those successes with you through-out this book—successes that can be yours as well.

In the pages that follow, we explain the unhealthy auto-immune processes that occur in the bodies of people who suffer with autoimmune diseases and discuss how those processes work in about twenty of the most common autoimmune diseases. Most importantly, we discuss how each of the treatment ap-proaches we use can alleviate or eliminate these conditions, and which remedies and lifestyle modifications you can use to help yourself and those you love.

If we just concentrated on eliminating the poisons that are in the human body, I believe we could successfully treat sufferers of autoimmune disease. I wrote this book as part of a major step in that direction. Too many people, especially women in their twen-ties, thirties, and forties, suffer with an autoimmune disorder. They come to me asking questions like: Why do I have this dis-ease? What is happening to my body? Why don't drugs and other conventional treatments make me feel better? Why don't doctors understand how to treat me? This book answers all those ques-tions. But perhaps the most important question is: Is there any-thing I can do to get better?

The answer is a resounding yes.

❖ HOW TO USE THIS BOOK

If you have or suspect you have an autoimmune condition, or you care about someone who does, you already know that it can be complex and confusing. In this book I try to make autoimmunity understandable and introduce you to treatment options. To get the most out of the book, I suggest the following approach.

First, read chapter 1 to discover exactly what we know about autoimmunity and how it works in the body. A basic understanding of the autoimmune process is essential if you hope to heal.

Next, read the beginning of chapter 2, up to "It's Test Time." Here's where you'll learn not only how autoimmunity is evaluated, but also what questions to ask when looking for a healthcare provider who understands how autoimmunity works and, more important, one who can help you. For now, you can skip the rest of chapter 2 until you need to refer back to it. Don't worry, I'll tell you when.

Each of chapters 3 through 10 gives a detailed description of the more common autoimmune conditions and how they can be treated. Turn to the chapter that describes your condition, or, if you've never been diagnosed, read the chapters that best match your symptoms. Use the information in these chapters in discussions with your doctor. You'll notice in each chapter that I discuss various tests that are done to diagnose each condition. Here's where you can turn back to chapter 2 and learn about each of these tests, if you're so moved. Perhaps you could share this chapter with your doctor as well, in order to help obtain a diagnosis.

Now you're ready for action. Chapters 11, 12, and 13 make up the cornerstone of my treatment approach to autoimmunity: biodetoxification, nutritional therapies, and immunotherapy. The treatment approaches explained in each of these chapters go to the roots of autoimmunity rather than just apply a bandage to the symptoms, like conventional medicine does. The treatments discussed include those only available through a knowledgeable physician, as well as actions you can take yourself, at home today. Everyone can benefit from the therapies covered in these three chapters.

Now it's up to you. Healing from autoimmunity takes time and dedication. This book is a toolbox: it contains informational and actionable tools. Open it and get to work!

Part I

---❖---

UNDERSTANDING
AUTOIMMUNITY

Chapter 1

What Is Autoimmunity?

You're alone, walking down a dark alley late at night. You're feeling strong and confident; there's a spring in your step, and you're striding with determination. Suddenly, out of nowhere, you're attacked from behind. Immediately you burst into action. You maneuver your way out of the stranglehold bear hug. You turn and quickly release a strategically placed kick. You send the invader to his knees, then pin him down just as reinforcements arrive to haul him away. And you didn't even break a sweat or a nail. You just did what you were trained and ready to do: protect yourself.

❖ THE IMMUNE SYSTEM

Protecting and preserving your health is exactly what your immune system is designed to do. Your immune system is a complex network of organs, glands, and special cells that encompass your entire body. Its purpose is to guard you against invaders that can harm you or compromise your body's ability to function in a healthy way. When your immune system is operating optimally—when all its components are healthy and alert—it can effectively fight off many different types of enemies, such as bacteria, viruses, parasites, and fungi, and the harmful effects of stress, household chemicals, secondhand smoke, pesticides, and food additives. Like a well-placed kick, the immune system fights back . . . and you win.

Unfortunately, people with an unhealthy immune system don't feel like their immune system is kicking back. Bea, a thirty-three-year-old mother of two girls, says she felt like she was the one being kicked. "I was exhausted and achy all the time," she says. "I felt like I was letting my husband and kids down because I was always too tired to go out. They were always going to the mall and to the park without me. I even missed my daughter's school play because I was too tired and depressed to leave the house."

"I was embarrassed to make any more excuses to my friends," says Lila, a forty-two-year-old graphic artist. "I had to make sure I was near a bathroom everywhere I went, because I never knew when the stomach cramps and diarrhea were going to hit me. It was safer to just stay home."

Bea and Lila are not alone. Millions of people are burdened with chronic, life-altering symptoms that often are manifestations of something gone awry with the immune system, causing it to turn against the body's cells. In Bea's case, the fourth doctor she saw diagnosed her with lupus before she came to see me. Lila found her way to the Edelson Center before getting a diagnosis, which we identified as Crohn's disease. Both women responded well to our treatment program.

What makes the immune system turn against the very body it inhabits? To understand this process, it helps to first know how the immune system works when it's healthy.

Meet the Players

The number and types of players involved in maintaining a healthy immune system are great—greater than can be described in detail here. But a basic knowledge of how they operate is important to understanding autoimmunity and any symptoms you may be experiencing. Therefore we explain the purpose of the main players below, since they are referred to again and again throughout this book.

Just as you would use a certain move to shrug off a bear hug and another to ward off an attack to your face, these players have specific moves that contribute to keeping your body functioning optimally. For example:

• **Thymus.** This is the master gland of the immune network. Located above the heart, it secretes various hormones that are responsible for regulating immune system functions. It also produces T-cells, which are another major player in immune system functioning (see below). The thymus is extremely susceptible to damage from stress, environmental toxins, infections, and chronic illness.

• **Skin and mucous membranes.** Your body's largest organ is the skin, which is also its first line of defense against intruders. Whenever it is compromised, say, with a cut, burn, abrasion, or puncture, there is an open door for disease-causing organisms to enter. The mucous membranes of the gastrointestinal tract, lungs, vagina, nose, mouth, and so on, are the body's "internal" skin, and are also a line of defense against invaders.

• **Bone marrow.** The center portion of bone is an area rich in blood vessels and other substances. It is here that many types of immune cells are manufactured.

• **Spleen.** This dark red organ, located on the left side of the upper abdominal region, manufactures lymphocytes (see below), attacks bacteria, and recycles damaged blood cells.

• **Lymph nodes.** These tiny, glandlike structures are found throughout the body, including under the arms, in the groin, and behind the ears. If you've ever had "swollen glands," what you actually had were inflamed lymph nodes. And the reason they were swollen is because the lymph nodes act as an inspection station for foreign substances, which they remove from the body's tissues. The lymph nodes prevent these substances from entering the bloodstream and finding their way to the organs.

• **Lymphatic system.** This network consists of lymph vessels, lymph nodes, and lymph, a thick fluid that is made up of fat and white blood cells. While the circulatory system is the transportation system for blood, the lymphatic system carries immune cells to parts of the body where they are needed.

• **Lymphocytes.** A type of white blood cell, lymphocytes are produced in the bone marrow and are found in the blood and in the spleen, lymph nodes, thymus, and other tissues. Lymphocytes perform four primary functions, all of which must work properly for a healthy immune system. They (1) recognize the invaders; (2) prepare a line of defense; (3) communicate with other essential immune system cells by producing cytokines (see below) and deploying them to act against the invaders; and (4) stop the action of the immune cells once their job is done. If any one of these steps goes awry, disease, including autoimmune conditions, can be the result. You'll be reading more about lymphocytes and their role in autoimmune conditions later. For now, here are some of the major types of lymphocytes and what they do:

➤ *B-lymphocytes (B-cells)* work along with T-cells (below) as the main line of defense for the body. They look for invading foreign proteins (called *antigens*) and "tag" or mark them with proteins called *antibodies*. This tag lets other immune cells know that an invader is in their midst so they can destroy it.

➤ *T-lymphocytes (T-cells)* reach maturity in the thymus and then circulate throughout both the lymphatic system and bloodstream. They initiate attacks against antigens, direct the fight, and then stop the destruction. T-cells are divided into several types. The ones we will concern ourselves with here are CD4 (helper T-cells), which act as cheerleaders and urge other immune cells to attack; and CD8 (suppressor cells), which make sure the helper T-cells don't overreact.

➤ *Natural killer cells* perform the dirty work. While B-cells simply "tag" the invaders, natural killer cells live up to their name and destroy them. They also produce hormonelike chemicals called *cytokines,* which are discussed below.

➤ *Macrophages* are known as the recyclers of the immune system, because they consume invading organisms, tumor cells, and dead red blood cells. They also produce cytokines.

• **Immunoglobulins.** Each B-lymphocyte produces a specific antibody, or immunoglobulin. There are five main types of immunoglobulins, which are named according to their presence in the blood: IgG, IgA, IgM, IgD, and IgE.

• **Interferon.** Interferons are a type of cytokine that you will read more about later in this book. There are several types of interferons, including alpha interferon and gamma interferon. For now, it's important that you know that interferons are powerful antiviral substances and that they are often used to treat cancer and hepatitis.

❖ COMMUNICATION IS THE KEY

These components, along with dozens of others, make up the immune system network. It's easy to see why with so many components, it would be easy for things to go wrong. For the most part, the immune system functions well because its cells communicate with each other, the brain, and other parts of the system. Their method of communication involves cytokines, hormonelike substances that transmit information among immune cells. Although immune cells don't have ears, they can detect minute changes in cytokine production, which in turn stimulates them to respond in certain ways, say, by launching an attack against certain invaders.

Some cytokines communicate not only with immune system cells but with nerve cells as well. These specialized cytokines, called interleukins, perform many critical and interesting tasks, some of which help support the idea of the mind-body relationship in medicine. Scientists know, for example, that the brain (a part of the nervous system) plays a key role in controlling our immune system and physical health. (In fact, the microglia in the brain is part of the immune system.) This is obvious when we consider the effects emotional stress and tension have on our body, causing headaches, neck and back pain, stomach distress, and many other symptoms. Thus, interleukins link the immune and nervous systems, a concept that will become more obviously important later when we discuss the effects of stress in people with autoimmune conditions.

Speaking of autoimmune conditions, now let's talk about when something goes wrong with immune system functioning.

❖ WHEN THINGS GO WRONG WITH THE IMMUNE SYSTEM

Let's go back to that dark alley. This time your head is down and you're dragging your feet. You've been working hard, you've been eating lots of processed fast foods, and you've been spending too much time in smoky nightclubs. This time when you're attacked, the mugger gets the best of you. Your immune cells fight back, but they're not as effective as they could be. So you get to spend a week feeling miserable with the flu, a stomach virus, or a bad cold.

No one's immune system operates perfectly all the time. It's virtually impossible to find a person who has never had a cold, suffered with the flu, had a toothache or ear infection, or gotten an infection from a cut or burn. But in most cases, the body's immune system eventually overcomes the invaders and the body returns to relative harmony.

Autoimmunity

Unfortunately, there are millions and millions of individuals whose immune systems do not respond normally to an attack. Instead of attacking foreign invaders with antibodies—substances produced by the immune system to fight invaders—the immune system components attack the body's own healthy cells—perhaps bones, joints, blood, brain, nerves, or other body parts—as if *they* were the enemy. When the immune system reacts in this way, it is producing *autoantibodies*—substances that attack healthy cells instead of foreign invaders. This situation is known as an *autoimmune response.*

More than eighty separate medical conditions have been recognized as being the result of an autoimmune response. Some of them are quite common; others are rare. In this book we concern ourselves with the more common conditions, including rheumatoid arthritis, lupus, multiple sclerosis, hypothyroidism (Hashimoto's thyroiditis), hyperthyroidism (Graves' disease), Crohn's disease, ulcerative colitis, type 1 diabetes, autism, chronic fatigue syndromes, ankylosing spondylitis, autoimmune hepatitis, autoimmune kidney disease, polymyositis, scleroderma, silicone immune toxicity syndrome, Sjögren's syndrome, and vasculitis.

On the surface, these conditions seem to be quite different. The symptoms of rheumatoid arthritis (inflamed, painful joints, limited mobility) are different from those common to Crohn's disease (chronic diarrhea, abdominal pain, fever). Yet the vast majority of autoimmune diseases share several important similarities:

- a genetic susceptibility for specific autoimmune conditions. It is unknown how many people have a genetic predisposition for autoimmunity and who will experience an autoimmune response; and
- environmental toxins that trigger the autoimmune response

It is these similarities, which we will discuss in the pages that follow, that have drawn me and other like-minded health professionals to successfully treat these autoimmune conditions using techniques not normally employed by conventional physicians. While conventional medicine simply treats the symptoms, we heal the body by going directly to the origins of the disease—the autoimmune response at the cellular level. To get a better understanding of how we do that, it's first important to understand why autoimmune conditions develop in the first place. The reason, I believe, is simple: direct damage and free-radical damage to cells from environmental toxins (heavy metals and chemicals).

Free Radicals

Free radicals are highly charged molecules that have an unpaired electron in their outer orbit. They are naturally present in the body and, in relatively small numbers, they perform essential tasks, such as destroying harmful bacteria. But when they increase in number, they can damage DNA, cell membranes, enzyme systems, and immune system functioning. (See box, "Oxidation [Free-Radical Damage] in a Nutshell.")

Because the natural order of the universe is toward balance, and free radicals are unbalanced molecules, they constantly steal electrons from other molecules, which in turn creates more free radicals. Unfortunately, our environment is increasingly becoming tainted with free radicals because of environmental toxins, such as pesticides, radiation, household chemicals, viruses, secondhand smoke, toxic waste, food additives, alcohol, and drugs. When these and other free radicals invade the body, they go on to create even more free radicals and thus have the potential to cause much damage to the body's cells. The damage that free radicals cause is called *oxidation.* (Such damage can be avoided or reduced if the body produces or takes in enough protective molecules called *antioxidants,* which will be discussed in chapter 12.)

Our bodies are constantly under attack by negative environmental factors, which means we are constantly fighting the effects of oxidation. Being in this state of *oxidative stress* is what makes us sick. For some people, for various reasons we will discuss later, free-radical damage and oxidative stress cause an autoimmune process and autoimmune disease.

Oxidation (Free-Radical Damage) in a Nutshell

The story of the autoimmune process is complex and not completely understood by scientists. However, to help you understand what may be happening in your body right now, here's a simplified explanation.

Have you ever seen metal turn rusty? A cut apple turn brown? These are examples of a chemical process called *oxidation*. On the surface we see the results of oxidation—the destruction of metal, the breakdown of fruit. But at a molecular level, electrons are being lost. That's where free radicals enter the picture, because they steal electrons from other molecules in your body. Free radicals are "oxidized" molecules.

Say free radical 1, a pesticide molecule, takes an electron from molecule 2. Molecule 2 is damaged and is transformed into free radical 2. Then free radical 2 takes an electron from molecule 3, which then becomes free radical 3, and so on. A pattern of cell destruction has begun.

Say molecule 2 was a normal nerve cell, thus removing the electron harms the cell. When normal cells are damaged by free radicals (oxidation) in people who have a predisposition (susceptibility) for autoimmunity, the immune system treats these now-damaged cells as invaders. This begins the autoimmune process, in which the body's immune system attacks the body's own cells, which it believes are invaders, causing the many symptoms seen in autoimmune diseases, such as fatigue, chronic pain, digestive problems, and muscle aches (see chapters 3–10).

Free radicals may also damage the DNA in cells that are part of the immune control function. There is a theory that says when free radicals damage the DNA in immune response cells that are responsible for fighting invaders, it also triggers an autoimmune response.

The bottom line is this: environmental toxins are all around us, and they stimulate the production of free radicals, which can cause oxidative damage to any kind of cell, be it muscle, nerve, liver, kidney, heart, brain, and so on, and cause autoimmune disease.

The Autoimmune Process

When the immune system is operating properly, it identifies, attacks, and eliminates foreign or invader cells. That's because the immune system components can correctly identify the difference between self-cells—those that are part of your body—and those that are not. Each of the self-cells is encoded with a tag, like a social security number, called the human leukocyte antigen (HLA). The HLA lets the immune system know that these self-antigens belong to the body.

Sometimes, however, the identification process goes awry. This can happen if normal self-cells are damaged or changed by free radicals so that the immune system now treats them as invaders. It can also happen when some lymphocytes become sensitized against self-cells (which is not unusual) and are not suppressed by other lymphocytes (which normally occurs). The reason these two situations can occur is not completely understood. However, scientists generally believe that environmental toxins can damage or alter self-cells and thus trigger an autoimmune process in people who are susceptible to autoimmunity (see box, "Oxidation [Free-Radical Damage] in a Nutshell," and "Genetics," below). In my practice I have found that environmental toxins—most toxic chemicals, lead, mercury, and nickel—are a causative ingredient in nearly all auto-immune conditions I have treated.

Autoimmune Process versus Autoimmune Disease

The autoimmune process typically becomes identified as an auto-immune disease when the free radicals have focused their attack on one or more specific cell types or organ systems in the body. For example, if the self-attack occurs in the joints and causes swelling, inflammation, and pain, these are symptoms of rheuma-toid arthritis. Individuals who experience DNA damage in the pancreas can develop type 1 diabetes. Individuals who have sys-temic lupus erythematosus (SLE) typically have several different tissues and organ systems involved, including the skin, nervous system, and heart tissue.

In my approach to treating people who have an autoimmune condition, I zero in on the autoimmune process, not the disease. I don't believe it is necessary to "label" the autoimmune disease in order to treat the patient, because what's important is to address the cause, and that cause, in my experience, is the same for nearly every case of autoimmune disease: environmental toxins.

I don't mean to sound as if autoimmune disorders are a snap to identify and treat. They are not—not for me nor for any other practitioner who takes on the challenge. Yet there are detailed, comprehensive steps that can be taken to deal with and success-fully treat the individuals who have these often debilitating con-ditions. And that is the focus of much of the rest of this book.

Autoimmune Disease Summary: Do You Have These Symptoms?

Researchers have identified more than eighty different auto-immune disorders, yet they all seem to share one characteristic: they are caused by free-radical damage. Free radicals damage normal self-cells, causing the immune system to perceive them as invaders in susceptible individuals. What triggers the molecular free-for-all in each susceptible individual and the disorder that will result from it, however, differs among people.

Here's a brief overview of autoimmune diseases. As you read through it, see if you identify with any of the symptoms or diseases. If you do, or you'd like to learn more about any of the conditions, you can find details in chapters 3 through 10.

SYMPTOMS

Although symptoms vary widely among all the different auto-immune disorders, they tend to share some very nonspecific ones, including:

- Fatigue
- Tire easily
- Fever (low-grade)
- Dizziness
- Malaise (generally not feeling well)

MOST COMMON AUTOIMMUNE DISEASES

• **Chronic fatigue and immune dysfunction syndrome (CFIDS):** characterized by extreme fatigue that is often debilitating, plus dozens of other symptoms that can affect systems throughout the body, such as swollen lymph nodes, sore throat, short-term memory problems, and muscle pain. I want to make it clear that although CFIDS has characteristics of autoimmunity, it is not, in my opinion, a primary autoimmune disease. It is within that context that we discuss it in chapter 10.

• **Crohn's disease and ulcerative colitis:** characterized by chronic inflammation of the intestinal tract. Typical symptoms include chronic diarrhea, fatigue, fever, abdominal pain, and weight loss. Crohn's disease and ulcerative colitis are types of inflammatory bowel disease, not to be confused with irritable bowel syndrome (IBS), which is not an autoimmune condition. Irritable bowel syndrome is marked by alternating diarrhea and constipation, indigestion, heartburn, and intestinal gas.

• **Diabetes (type 1):** failure to produce insulin because of autoimmune attack on the islet cells (which produce insulin) of the pancreas. Approximately 800,000 people in the United States have type 1 diabetes, which typically first appears during the first twenty years of life. Symptoms of the disease include excessive thirst and hunger, frequent urination, fatigue, and weakness.

• **Graves' disease:** a thyroid condition characterized by hyperthyroidism (symptoms include nervousness, hypersensitivity to heat, palpitations, fatigue, increased appetite, weight loss, rapid heartbeat, insomnia, weakness), as well as one or more of the following: an enlarged thyroid, bulging eyeballs, tremor of fingers and muscles of the hands, increased metabolism, and other symptoms. Graves' disease occurs in response to autoantibodies that stimulate the TSH (thyroid-stimulating hormone) receptors in the thyroid (see "Autoimmune Thyroid Disease," in chapter 2).

• **Hashimoto's thyroiditis:** a condition in which the thyroid is enlarged. Thyroid function is suppressed because of a deficiency of thyroid secretion, prompted by autoantibodies that attack thyroglobulin and thyroid peroxidase enzymes. It is the most common cause of hypothyroidism. Symptoms include dull facial expression; puffiness around the eyes; coarse, dry hair; coarse, dry, scaly, and thick skin; constipation; and enlarged heart.

• **Lupus:** characterized by inflammation of tissues throughout the body, including the muscles, connective tissue, heart, eyes, and brain, caused by autoantibodies that attack cells' DNA. This disease affects ten times more women than men, with symptoms that include achy joints, fever, arthritis, severe fatigue, facial rash, and myocardial problems, among many others. People with lupus often experience a roller-coaster effect, with periods during which symptoms are pronounced, followed by remission, only for the cycle to repeat again and again.

• **Multiple sclerosis:** the result of a delayed hypersensitivity response involving T-cells, leading to destruction of the myelin sheaths that protect the nerves. About twice as many women as men get the disease. Symptoms of multiple sclerosis can vary widely and depend on where in the body the myelin has been damaged. Therefore, damage to the motor nerves may result in vision problems, muscle weakness, and bowel and bladder difficulties, while deterioration of the sensory nerves can cause tingling and numbness in different parts of the body.

• **Rheumatoid arthritis:** T-cells and cytokines attack the joints, which causes inflammation and destruction of the synovial membranes in the joints, resulting in pain, tenderness, stiffness, and swelling. Onset of the disease is usually between twenty and forty-five years, and about 75 percent of the 2.5 million Americans with rheumatoid arthritis are women.

Autism: An Autoimmune Disease?

Autism is a condition characterized by psychiatric disturbances, speech and language problems, sensory abnormalities, cognitive difficulties, and unusual behaviors. It is estimated to affect about 1 to 2 of every 500 children in the United States. Categorizing autism as an autoimmune condition is controversial, but it is an avenue I believe should be explored, and is being studied by a few researchers. In my practice, I have found that 50 percent of the children who have autism also have evidence of autoimmunity: they have autoantibodies to proteins of the central nervous system, as are seen in other autoimmune disorders. Also, most children with autism also have specific immune system problems, such as food and inhalant allergies, and decreased natural killer cell activity, both common in autoimmune disorders. Although categorizing autism as a condition with autoimmune components is controversial, it is, in my opinion and in the opinions of researchers who are investigating the autism–autoimmune connection, well worth researching further, especially as this condition has reached epidemic proportions. For these reasons, the autism–autoimmune connection is explored in chapter 3.

❖ THE ROLE OF ENVIRONMENTAL TOXINS IN THE AUTOIMMUNE PROCESS

Although environmental toxins are not the only cause of the autoimmune process, I don't think I have treated an autoimmune patient who has not been toxic. During the many years I have treated people with autoimmune process conditions, most patients have been either completely or significantly relieved of their symptoms once toxins were removed from their body—patients like Leonard, a bright twenty-one-year-old man whose life was being devastated by Crohn's disease. Gradual removal of the lead and mercury found in his body, along with supportive therapies, completely changed his life within months of starting treatment. His story and others, told in chapters 3 through 10, are examples of the role of environmental toxins in the autoimmune process, and how removing them provides people with the relief for which they've been searching.

We live in a toxic world. That statement is not meant to scare you, but to make you realize that the problem exists, that environmental toxins are making hundreds of millions of people sick around the world, and to increase your awareness of the fact that toxins surround you every day. Consider this: an estimated 25 percent of Americans have some form of heavy metal poisoning, including mercury, lead, arsenic, cadmium, aluminum, and nickel. These materials are associated with dozens of different medical disorders and symptoms. For decades we didn't think or worry about these and other environmental pollutants. Very few people spoke out about their potential dangers. After all, we were being promised a better world through chemicals. Little did most people know that many of those chemicals would prove to be damaging and even deadly to humans.

Fortunately, more and more researchers and physicians are recognizing that heavy metals and chemicals that are present in our everyday environment—at home, at school, in parks and playgrounds—are at the core of the increase in the number of people who are affected by autoimmune disorders. In an article published in the *Journal of Toxicology and Environmental Health,* the authors had this to say about pesticide use:

> Because of the wide use of pesticides for domestic and industrial purposes the evaluation of the immunotoxic

[poison to the immune system] effects is of major concern for public health. The association between autoimmune diseases and pesticide exposure has been suggested. A potential risk for the immune system should [be considered], especially . . . in compromised patients [such as] children and the elderly. Epidemiological studies of diseases related to immunosuppression or autoimmunity—lupus erythematosus, rheumatoid arthritis—are warranted.

Consider one of the most common poisons to which we are exposed: mercury. It can be found in our drinking water, in the air we breathe, in our dental fillings, and in the fish we eat. Once it is in the body, mercury affects both the immune and nervous systems by damaging neurons and the transmission of signals in the brain, causing symptoms such as loss of sensation, vision problems, muscle weakness, incoordination, loss of memory, chronic fatigue, and tremors. You may recognize these symptoms as being associated with several common autoimmune diseases, such as multiple sclerosis and lupus. Mercury toxicity has also been linked with rheumatoid arthritis, Alzheimer's disease, autism, depression, attention deficit hyperactivity disorder, and many other conditions. Can we say with 100 percent certainty that mercury is at the root of these conditions? No. But mercury is an extremely dangerous toxin, and we have compelling evidence that it contributes to many medical conditions.

Making the Toxin–Autoimmune Connection

It's important to keep in mind that establishing the link between environmental toxins and autoimmunity is pioneering work. Most researchers and physicians have not yet jumped onto the bandwagon, but those who have, like myself, are exploring an important and complex frontier. Why don't we have research results that show a clear cause-and-effect between toxins and various autoimmune conditions in humans? Because it would be unethical to conduct controlled scientific studies in which we inject people with mercury or other toxins and then observe them over a period of years to see how their immune system responds and destroys cells and tissues throughout the body. That's why the vast majority of research has been done using animal models and cell cultures.

Studies have shown that exposure to heavy metals such as mercury, cadmium, and lead can be linked to the autoimmune process and that environmental toxins such as trichloroethylene (a common industrial solvent to which approximately 3.5 million workers are exposed in the United States) have been associated with the development of the autoimmune diseases scleroderma, autoimmune hepatitis, lupus, and systemic sclerosis. Dozens of common chemicals found readily in your environment, including benzene, hydrocarbons, insecticides, ozone, and formaldehyde, have been shown to elicit toxic responses of the immune system.

Heavy Metals:
Doing Heavy Damage to the Body

When heavy metal molecules get into the body, they create free radicals and disturb cell membranes and enzyme activities. For example, metals can bind to cell membranes and alter the cells' ability to perform their specific tasks, and cause cell death. Depending on people's genetic predisposition for effectively eliminating toxins from the body, different individuals may tolerate more or less exposure to toxic metals before showing negative effects such as an autoimmune process or an allergic response. Genetics apparently determines which part(s) of the body the toxins will attack.

Although researchers do conduct experiments in animals, we also have many human anecdotal reports that link toxins and autoimmune disorders. Few things speak truer than success. In my practice, *I have repeatedly shown that removing the toxins from people who have an autoimmune process running rampant in their body brings relief.* You will read about some of these individuals in chapters 3 through 10, as well as discussions on ways to remove those toxins in chapter 11.

❖ OTHER FACTORS AND THE AUTOIMMUNE PROCESS

Certainly not everyone who is exposed to environmental toxins—and that's nearly everyone on the planet—develops an autoimmune disease. So what makes some people more susceptible than others?

Genetics

Genetics works hand in hand with environmental factors in autoimmunity. It is generally believed that people who develop an autoimmune condition are genetically susceptible to do so. What is especially interesting about autoimmune conditions is that a family history of *any* autoimmune disorder generally increases one's risk of getting *the same or another* autoimmune condition.

(As you'll see in chapters 3–10, the degree of risk varies with the specific autoimmune disease.) Thus, what people inherit is not the likelihood to get a *particular* autoimmune disease but the tendency for the *autoimmune process,* or autoimmunity. Our understanding of the genetic influence in autoimmunity is still in its infancy, but generally it is believed that genetic factors contribute about one-third to one-half of the risk for most autoimmune conditions.

For example, if your grandmother has rheumatoid arthritis, you have hypothyroidism, and your daughter has lupus, each of you inherited the tendency for autoimmunity. However, each of these conditions has its own unique genes that are associated with the disease, so each of you has a different manifestation of autoimmunity.

Diet

Diet is an important factor in autoimmunity because poor nutrition compromises the immune system, and a compromised system can't fight back effectively. If you have a tendency for autoimmunity, a poor diet is your ticket for trouble.

Unless you are one of the few who eat a totally organic, whole foods diet, which is virtually free of environmental contaminants, you probably follow the Standard American Diet, or SAD, which it is. This nutritionally poor diet consists primarily of processed foods, meat and dairy products tainted with hormones and other drugs, lots of sugary items, alcohol, and few fresh fruits and vegetables. It is a menu for disaster and a compromised immune system.

SAD lacks sufficient servings of fruits and vegetables, which are rich sources of antioxidants, the front line of defense against free radicals. The hormones, steroids, and other drugs found in most meats and dairy products can be toxic to the body—

environmental toxins, if you will, that can cause the formation of free radicals, which in turn damage your cells. Processed foods not only have insufficient amounts of nutrients, but they also contain immune-system-damaging substances, such as sugars, hydrogenated fats and oils (which contain trans fatty acids), artificial sweeteners, and artificial colors, preservatives, and flavors. In short, these are not whole, natural foods and so are foreign to the body. (See chapter 12 for more on diet.)

Stress

With so much emphasis today on the mind-body connection in health, it's no surprise that stress is a major factor in immune system functioning in general and in the autoimmune process in particular. In *The Stress of Life*, Dr. Hans Selye wrote, "If a microbe [invader] is in or around us all the time and yet causes no disease until we are exposed to stress, what is the cause of the illness, the microbe or the stress?" His answer is that both contribute to the illness, and it appears that this is true. You have probably experienced this effect. When you're overtired, overworked, and not eating properly, your immune system is compromised. Studies have shown that stress can suppress the immune system and make you more susceptible to illness. Thus you're much more likely to contract a cold or flu that is circulating through your office than if you are well rested, eating nutritionally balanced meals, and putting in an average workweek.

Unmanaged or mismanaged stress is just one risk factor for the development of major disease. It certainly is a factor in the biggest killers in the United States, heart disease and cancer, as well as in lupus, Crohn's disease, depression, headache and migraine, hypertension, and various other disorders.

*   *   *

Noel R. Rose, M.D., Ph.D., of Johns Hopkins University and chairperson of the American Autoimmune Related Disease Association National Scientific Advisory Board, says that while genetics is one-half of the story behind autoimmune disease, "we're beginning to define the other half of the story, the environmental half. It is going to be, I think, an equally fascinating chapter in the saga of autoimmune disease in the next decade." I believe he is right, and I want to share with you what we know so far about that chapter—and how it can help anyone who has an autoimmune disorder—in the pages ahead.

❖ TREATING AUTOIMMUNITY

Remember the weed and lawn analogy I used in the introduction, in which I said if you want to get rid of the weeds you must do more than just mow down the tops and expect the weeds not to grow back? If you have an autoimmune condition and you go to a conventional doctor, she or he will mow your lawn: you'll be given drugs that will knock down your symptoms, but the roots of your disease will still be strong. This approach offers only temporary relief at best.

So I'd like to close this chapter on a hopeful note, and much of that hope lies in the cornerstones of my three-pronged treatment approach—biodetoxification, nutritional therapies, and immunotherapy, discussed in chapters 11, 12, and 13, respectively. This method attacks the roots of autoimmunity. I've found that by combining various elements of these three treatment disciplines, chosen, of course, based on an individual's needs, I can successfully guide people back to health. *Elements of all three are necessary for successful healing.*

In biodetoxification, for example, we rid the body of heavy metals and other toxins that trigger autoimmunity, using techniques such as high-temperature saunas and chelation. Biodetox-ification must be supported by excellent nutrition, so I devise a supplement program that addresses each person's deficiencies and imbalances. My nutritional therapy approach also looks at a very common condition in autoimmunity—leaky gut syndrome. Most people who have this syndrome—in which heavy metals and other toxins damage the intestinal lining and allow harmful substances to enter the bloodstream—don't even realize it. You'll learn what you can do to correct this disorder in chapter 12.

The third critical cornerstone of my treatment approach is immunotherapy. Treatments in this category modulate, or har-monize, the immune system. In autoimmunity, in which the immune system is overactive, I use modulators that suppress overactivity, such as transfer factor, thymus extracts, and ozone therapy. Immunotherapy works along with biodetoxification and nutritional therapy to promote healing.

Before you delve into the various autoimmune diseases and treatments, I'd like you to read the beginning of the following chapter. The road to healing autoimmunity is not one you should walk alone. Although you can arm yourself with information and adopt a healing lifestyle—all of which we help you with in this book—aligning yourself and working with a knowledgeable healthcare professional is critical. In the next chapter you'll learn how to find such an individual and the questions you should ask to make sure you're getting the best guidance available.

Chapter 2

The Evaluation: How Do I Know If I Have an Autoimmune Disease?

Uncovering the intricate workings of the autoimmune process in any given individual can be likened to several things: a juicy detective story, assembling a 3-D jigsaw puzzle, or searching for clues to buried treasure. Although the process of evaluating a person's autoimmune disorder cannot be classified as "fun," especially for the person who is suffering with the symptoms, it is definitely a process of discovery and, forgive me, adventure.

That's because the human body is an incredibly complex structure, with its myriad components each having specialized, often interdependent tasks. And when things go awry as they do in an autoimmune process, the challenge is to try to make it right—to bring balance back to the body and relief to the individual.

As with all journeys, the one of discovering the autoimmune process begins with the first step: evaluating people's signs, symptoms, and complaints (see box, "Sign or Symptom?"), and then choosing tests and procedures that will reveal what is happening at the cellular level to cause those problems. In this chapter I explain how I discover the autoimmune process in individuals who come to me for help.

A few words before we begin. The majority of doctors do not use the evaluation methods I do. Most physicians are interested in "defining" or naming the condition so they can treat symptoms. Their "adventure," and ultimately that of their patients, goes something like this: you go to a doctor (or two or three) complaining, for example, of fatigue, depression, insomnia, muscle aches, fever, and feeling lousy. The doctor runs a bunch of tests, says he can't find anything wrong, and gives you a prescription to help you sleep and improve your mood. Or the doctor runs some blood tests, says they look good, but gives you a prescription for your aches and pains—"probably a touch of arthritis"—and says you'll be fine. Or the doctor says your blood pressure is high and that you should lose some weight. He gives you some blood pressure medication and sends you home. Or . . . you get the picture. Your symptoms are being treated, but no one has done a comprehensive evaluation or looked at the whole picture to locate the root of your problem.

My goal, however, is to find the cause and origins of the complaint at the cellular level so we can eliminate the basic problem. There are some doctors like myself—practicing a new and unique field of medicine called clinical molecular medicine—who use some or many of the techniques discussed here. Clinical molecular medicine integrates environmental medicine, applied immunology (the study of immune system function), toxicology (the study of toxins that may cause illness), free-radical medicine (the study of the effects of free-radical damage), and clinical nutritional biochemistry (the study of chemical processes at the cellular level). In this chapter we explain how to find doctors who practice the pioneering field of clinical molecular medicine.

The tests explained in this chapter are but a few of the hundreds that can be used to evaluate people who have autoimmune symptoms. We have included only some of the ones I most commonly use. You don't need to read about these tests right now. Once you turn to the chapters that discuss the various autoimmune conditions (chapters 3 through 10), you'll be referred back to this chapter to learn more about the tests used to diagnose those conditions.

Now, before you leave this chapter and turn to the ones that discuss various autoimmune conditions, learn more about how to find a doctor who can help you. First, I'll tell you how I approach new patients and the types of questions I ask them. Then, because everyone can't come to see me, I offer some guidelines on how to find a doctor who can help you. What questions should you ask of prospective doctors? What questions should he or she be asking *you*?

❖ GETTING TO KNOW YOU

Each patient is a unique individual with a personal and family history, environmental history, symptoms, and lifestyle that make a defining impact on that person's health and autoimmune process. When you visit a doctor for the first time, you can expect to fill out a page or two about your personal and family history and check off your symptoms on a list, and then undergo a physical examination based on your complaints.

To get to the core of an autoimmune process, I believe doctors need to go much further and deeply explore an individual's environmental exposure. Where on a conventional doctor's history questionnaire will you find questions about your exposure to chemicals or pesticides? Do any of them ever ask about the types of chemical exposures your parents had? Do they ask what type of chemicals you use in your home? Have you ever been asked if you live near a power generating station or microwave tower, whether you bleach or dye your hair, or if you have your clothes dry-cleaned?

The truth is, I have found that environmental factors—substances not only in the air and water but also in our food—have a tremendous and critically important impact on health and the immune system. If we, as doctors, neglect to explore those influences, we are, in my view, essentially practicing poor medicine and committing an injustice to the people who come to us looking for help. As doctors, we need to have all the information we can so that we can make informed evaluations of our patients.

That's why I use a Comprehensive Medical History Evaluation Questionnaire as part of my evaluation process. Without it, I believe my patients would be cheated out of the opportunity to get the best care and a chance for a resolution to their health problems. The information gathered from that questionnaire (sample questions are given below), along with a person's symptoms and results of a physical examination, allows me to better identify the autoimmune process that is taking place. Then I can choose the most appropriate tests and the best treatment course for that person.

Sign or Symptom?

Yes, they are different. Signs are objective markers that your physician looks for when he or she examines you. If she notices that your throat is red and swollen, that's a sign. It can be seen and measured. Symptoms, however, are sensations or feelings that you report. In this case, you would probably report throat pain, but can that pain be accurately measured? Pain is subjective; every person experiences and reports it differently.

❖ THE QUESTIONNAIRE

Two to three pages versus fifty: that's the physical difference between the size of the questionnaire the vast majority of doctors use when you visit their office and the one I use. My Comprehensive Questionnaire covers you from head to toe; I like to say that I leave no cell unturned. Although fifty pages sounds daunting, patients find that the questionnaire is not only painless (no poking or prodding involved), but also enlightening. It is rewarding to piece together how influences from patients' past and current environments, along with a very detailed inquiry into symptoms and reactions, can uncover a wealth of information about a person's health. When we are done with the questions, we have created a solid picture of the individual, and we have a better idea of how to approach treatment.

Below are some sample questions from the hundreds that make up the Comprehensive Medical History Evaluation Questionnaire. Before you look them over, I'd like to explain something. If you have symptoms of autoimmunity and you find yourself answering yes to even a few of these questions, it is likely that my approach to treating autoimmunity will help you. Affirmative answers to questions concerning exposure to environmental toxins are especially revealing; however, I cannot tell you that if you answer yes to a specific number of questions, it means that you definitely have an autoimmune condition. Each person's answers are weighed individually and considered along with a physical examination and the results of any tests that may be indicated.

- Is your skin sensitive to: sun, fabrics, detergents, or other products?
- Have you ever had allergy tests? If yes, when and what type?
- In the past thirty days, how many times have you consumed fish or fish products? (This concerns mercury exposure.)
- Have you been exposed to any of the following items (this concerns mercury exposure): mascara, skin-lightening creams, laxatives, calamine lotion, contact lens solution, latex paints, fabric softeners, floor waxes and polishes, wood preservatives, tattooing, batteries, fungicides for lawns?
- Have you taken tetracyclines or other antibiotics for acne for one month or more?
- Have you ever taken prednisone or other cortisone drugs for less than two weeks? More than two weeks?
- Have you ever taken birth control pills?
- If you are experiencing fatigue:

  ➤ Has it lasted for six months and been continuous or relapsing?
  ➤ Has any physician evaluated you to attempt to find out the cause?
  ➤ Does your fatigue begin when you awaken in the A.M.?
  ➤ Are you able to exercise?
  ➤ Does your fatigue interfere with your work, household activities, eating, reading, hobbies, sex?

- Have you ever had athlete's foot, ringworm, jock itch, or other fungal infections of the nails or skin?
- Do you know of any landfills near your home?
- Have you checked your house for radon?
- Do you work in a modern office with computers and copiers?
- Have you noticed mold or mildew in your home?
- Do you have fillings in your teeth? What type?
- Do you have indoor plants? How many?
- Do you regularly have your house treated for insects?
- Is there a power transformer near your home?
- Would you be sick if you had to try on newly dry-cleaned clothing or wear clothing that has been cleaned in chlorine bleach?
- Would you be sick if you had to swim for twenty minutes in a chlorinated pool?
- Do you experience any of the following signs and symptoms (characteristic of adrenal insufficiency): fatigue, irritability, depression, apprehension, weakness, headache, palpitations, cravings for salt and/or sweets, tender lymph nodes in neck, thin dry skin, scant perspiration, sparse hair, inability to concentrate, poor memory, frustration, pain in the upper back and neck, back pain, postural hypotension (low blood pressure when rising from a seated or lying position)?
- Have you ever experienced a rash from cosmetics or metals?
- As an infant and child, were you bothered by any of the following: certain foods, poor appetite, constipation, colic, headaches, gas, stomachaches, hives, rash, leg aches, eczema, night sweats, diarrhea, behavior problems, vomiting, fussiness?
- Is there a family history of allergies or food intolerance?
- Have you ever had a negative reaction to the following: dental anesthesia, other anesthesia, iodines, X-ray contrast media, tetanus or other vaccinations?

- What do you mostly eat: fresh, canned, frozen, or packaged food?

❖ FINDING A CLINICAL MOLECULAR MEDICINE PHYSICIAN

Clinical molecular medicine is an innovative and unique approach to medicine, because it integrates factors that are so critical in affecting our health in today's complicated and toxic world. Those factors include:

- Environmental medicine, which looks at the effects of the environment on human health
- Free-radical medicine, which explores the effects of free-radical damage on the body
- Applied immunology, the study of how the immune system functions
- Toxicology, an exploration of toxins that may cause illness
- Clinical nutritional biochemistry, which looks at the relationship between chemical processes and cell functioning

Physicians like myself who practice this medical approach are less concerned about naming an illness and more interested in identifying the basic mechanisms behind it. That means we look deep into the molecular workings of the body—inside the cells—to find what is not functioning properly. Then we use molecular methods to treat and prevent disease, imbalance, or dysfunction in the body. Those molecular methods include some of the things you'll read about in this book, such as biodetoxification, nutritional therapy, and immunotherapy (see chapters 11 through 13).

How do you find a clinical molecular physician? Currently, few doctors in the United States practice this type of medicine.

To see if there's one in your area, here are some of the questions you need to ask prospective candidates:

- Do you use biodetoxification methods in your practice, and what are they? (See chapter 11.)
- Do you use chelation for removal of heavy metals?
- Do you take an extensive environmental history of patients on their first visit?
- Do you do a thorough evaluation of dietary habits?
- Is nutritional supplementation an integral part of your treatment approach for autoimmune disorders?
- Do you test for food sensitivities and allergies?
- Do you thoroughly evaluate to seek the root cause of chronic disease?
- Do you use immunotherapy, and what approaches do you use? (See chapter 13.)

Ideally, you need a doctor who answers yes to all of these questions. A positive response to just one or two will not connect you with a clinical molecular physician. Interested individuals may contact the Edelson Center for help in locating such physicians. Our contact information can be found in the "Closing Comments."

There are also some general questions and factors to consider when choosing a physician. Here are some questions and guidelines:

• Where did the doctor attend medical school? You can verify a doctor's training and certification status at the American Medical Association's Physician Select, at www.ama-assn.org/aps/amahg.htm. This service is free.

• Is the doctor board certified? You can find out if a doctor is truly certified in a certain field if you contact the American Board of Medical Specialties Certified Doctor Verification Service. This is a free service and is available at www.abms.org/newsearch.asp.

• How many years has the doctor been practicing?

• Has the doctor ever been convicted of fraud, or has a state disciplinary board ever taken action against him or her? You can find out by contacting Medi-Net (www.askmedi.com), which has access to information on more than 900,000 licensed doctors in the United States. There is a fee for this service (under $20).

• Most state medical boards also list the names of disciplined doctors on their Web sites. See the Public Citizen Health Research Group, which has links to each state's Web site. This service is free (www.citizen.org/hrg/publications/1506.htm).

• What health insurance does the doctor accept?

• Does the doctor respond to patients' e-mail questions?

• Does the doctor respond to calls at night or on weekends?

• Does the doctor practice alone or in a group? If the doctor is unavailable, will you be referred to another doctor in the group?

• Is the doctor's office conveniently located, and are the office hours convenient for you?

❖ IT'S TEST TIME

Based on a patient's symptoms, the results of the physical examination, and the information I gather from the questionnaire, I choose the tests I believe will best identify the processes that are occurring at a molecular level—the "guts" of the problem. Here are some of the more common tests I consider using when a patient comes to me with autoimmune symptoms. These are but a representative listing and by no means the entire arsenal of tests available.

This chapter contains brief explanations of some of the tests I often use for patients who come to the Edelson Center. These tests can be ordered by your doctor, and in many cases they are covered by insurance, depending on your plan. You will see these tests mentioned throughout chapters 3 through 10, where I discuss how I evaluate and treat each condition. If you'd like, you may now move on to the chapter that specifically discusses your autoimmune disorder, then refer back to this chapter as needed to review the specific tests and what they can tell you.

❖ SPECIFIC TESTS FOR ORGAN SYSTEM COMPLAINTS

I may choose to conduct tests in these categories based on an individual's signs and symptoms, to determine the extent of damage or abnormality.

Gastrointestinal Symptoms

• **CDSA (comprehensive digestive stool analysis).** A stool sample is taken and evaluated to determine the status of the gastrointestinal tract. It can pinpoint imbalances and provide clues about symptoms. For example, it can detect the presence of various microorganisms that are known to cause inflammation, diarrhea, maldigestion, malabsorption, and other problems common to people who have an autoimmune disorder.

• **Lactulose mannitol challenge.** This test is used to gauge intestinal permeability. Intestinal permeability refers to the integrity of the walls of the intestines. The lining of the intestines not only absorbs nutrients but also helps keep out invading organisms. When this lining is attacked by things like bacteria, yeast, NSAIDs (nonsteroidal anti-inflammatory drugs like ibuprofen), alcohol, heavy metals, chemicals, and free radicals, it is damaged and loses its integrity. That leaves the way open for invaders to get in and cause inflammation, infection, and a condition known as "leaky gut syndrome." This is a term you want to remember. Why? According to Zoltan P. Rona, M.D., M.S., an authority on leaky gut syndrome, "The leaky gut syndrome is almost always associated with autoimmune disease and reversing autoimmune disease depends on healing the lining of the gastrointestinal tract." Unfortunately, about 30 percent of people who have leaky gut don't know it because they have no symptoms, thus it may not be detected unless an astute physician tests for it. (See chapter 12 for more information on leaky gut syndrome and how it is treated.) In the lactulose mannitol challenge study, patients swallow two sugars—lactulose and mannitol. Because these sugars are not metabolized in the body, their presence at high levels in urine may indicate leaky gut syndrome.

Hormonal System

• **DHEA levels.** DHEA (dehydroepiandrosterone) is a naturally occurring hormone that is produced and secreted by the adrenal glands. It is sometimes called the "mother hormone" because it is a precursor (something that precedes another) to many other hormones, including the sex hormones. Although levels of DHEA naturally decline as people age, women with lupus or rheumatoid arthritis have lower levels of this hormone than healthy individuals of the same age. DHEA levels can be measured in saliva, blood, and urine.

• **Sex hormone levels.** Levels of testosterone, estrogen, and progesterone can be measured in blood, saliva, and urine, and are important to identify because they can affect immune cell function and activity. Generally, high levels of testosterone and progesterone are suppressive to the immune system, and estrogen modulates it. The symptoms associated with some autoimmune disorders change with the natural fluctuations in estrogen and progesterone, such as those that occur during the menstrual cycle, menopause, and pregnancy. In some cases, the onset of an auto-immune disorder coincides with pregnancy or menopause. Examples include autoimmune thyroid disorders (Hashimoto's thyroiditis and Graves' disease) and rheumatoid arthritis, whose symptoms generally improve during pregnancy (progesterone levels are elevated during pregnancy, and to a lesser degree so are estrogen levels) but return once the baby is born. Given that the majority of people who get autoimmune disorders are women, the role of sex hormones in autoimmunity is significant, although scientists have yet to identify the scope of their involvement.

Central Nervous System

• **Neurotransmitters.** Both blood (for platelet levels) and urine samples are taken to determine the levels of these molecules, which are necessary for brain functioning. Once a deficiency is identified, therapy can begin to restore them to normal levels.

• **Evoked potentials.** These tests measure the brain's response to certain stimuli in three areas: visual, auditory, and sensory. The tests are painless and involve applying small metal disks to the scalp using a gel. These allow the brain's responses to specific stimuli to be recorded. During an auditory evoked potential test, for example, a series of clicks are presented in each ear, one at a time. Evoked potentials are used for autism and sometimes for multiple sclerosis and other demyelinating disorders.

• **Electromyogram (EMG).** This test is used when individuals have muscle weakness, to determine whether it is caused by a muscle condition or a neurological disorder, such as multiple sclerosis or myasthenia gravis. It is performed by inserting a needle electrode through the skin into the muscle. The electrode transmits information back to a computer. You may then be asked to contract the muscle (bend your arm, for example), and the size, shape, and overall presence of the wave that appears on the screen indicates the ability of the muscle to respond to nervous stimulation. More than one electrode may need to be placed to get an accurate reading.

• **Nerve conduction velocity.** This test is used to diagnose nerve damage, and is often done along with an EMG. It involves the placement of electrodes on the skin (with patches, similar to those used for an electrocardiogram) at various sites. One electrode emits a very mild electrical impulse and stimulates the nerve. The other electrodes record the amount of electrical activity. Abnormal findings indicate polymyositis or demyelinating disorders such as multiple sclerosis and myasthenia gravis.

• **Magnetic resonance imaging** (MRI). This noninvasive test provides a clear picture of various types of nerve tissue in the brain and a good indication of blood flow and the flow of cerebrospinal fluid. The procedure involves lying on a narrow table that is slid into a tunnel-like structure housing a scanner. The scanner creates a magnetic field around the body and sends radio waves to the tissues being studied. There is no radiation involved. MRI is useful for diagnosing demyelinating disorders, such as multiple sclerosis.

• **Electroencephalogram** (EEG). This test is used to detect disturbances that affect the brain. The procedure is painless. While you lie on a table or sit in a reclining chair, a technician applies electrodes to various sites on your scalp. The electrodes are connected by wires to a recording device, which converts the electrical signals from your brain into waves on a piece of paper. Abnormal findings may indicate the presence of multiple sclerosis.

Cardiovascular, Pulmonary, Genitourinary

Depending on the symptoms patients have when I interview and examine them, we may select various tests of their cardiovascular, pulmonary, or genitourinary systems. An echocardiogram, for example, may be indicated for someone who has lupus, because myocardial problems are common in this disorder.

❖ TOXICITY EVALUATION

• **Heavy metal challenge.** This evaluation is done by giving three different chelators (substances that bind to heavy metals) to the patient: an intravenous infusion of DMPS; an oral or suppository DMSA; and a dose of EDTA by intravenous infusion (see chapter 11). These chelators are administered during the same session, and the amounts given depend on the person's weight. Urine samples are collected from the individual over the next twelve hours and the levels of heavy metals are analyzed. Urine rather than blood samples is used, because heavy metals tend to clear quickly from blood. This evaluation is also used to monitor how effective treatment is and how long it must continue. Although this evaluation tests for thirty different toxic elements, the ones that are most commonly found are mercury, tin, cobalt, titanium, lead, nickel, arsenic, and cadmium.

• **Toxic (blood) chemistry studies.** A blood test that can detect levels of toxic chemicals, such as pesticides (DDT, DDE), toluene, hexane, pentane, tetrachloroethylene, formaldehyde, benzene, and dozens of other chemicals that can cause the creation of free radicals in the body. There are more than a dozen different tests (or panels) available, and each panel tests for a different category of chemical. I decide which test(s) to give based on the results of the Comprehensive Medical History Evaluation Questionnaire and symptoms.

❖ INFECTIOUS ORGANISM EVALUATION

A procedure called PCR (polymerase chain reaction) is highly effective in the detection of organisms such as bacteria (e.g., chlamydia), viruses (e.g., Epstein-Barr virus), fungi, and yeast (e.g., candida). It is a technique in which specific fragments of DNA are rapidly copied. This allows scientists to identify organisms from infinitely small amounts of tissue, blood, hair, or other substances. (This method is also used in crime labs to identify DNA samples.) Within minutes, PCR can amplify a single DNA molecule into billions of molecules. PCR is also used to detect mycoplasmas, microorganisms that are even smaller than bacteria.

It is controversial as to whether mycoplasmas or other organisms cause autoimmunity. It may be that if the immune system is suppressed, mycoplasmas may grow as a result of the suppression, and autoimmunity could then be a result of that process. This relationship has not yet been determined.

❖ DETOXIFICATION EVALUATION

These tests are done to determine the efficiency of a person's liver detoxication process.

Phase 1 and 2 Liver Detoxication Profile

This test assesses the function of the liver and its ability to process and eliminate toxins from the body, and evaluates the risk of free-radical damage caused by impaired liver function. The liver detoxication profile is an invaluable tool in assessing anyone who has heavy metal and/or chemical toxicity. The test is given by taking low doses of caffeine, aspirin, and acetaminophen and then collecting saliva, blood, and urine samples. The liver detoxication profile is unique in that it is the only test that can evaluate the functional capacity of the liver during both phases of detoxication: phase 1 and phase 2.

A brief explanation of phase 1 and phase 2 liver detoxication will help you better understand why biodetoxification is so critical to healing from heavy metal and chemical toxicity.

During phase 1, some chemical toxins that have been carried to the liver in the blood and lymph are transformed into substances that can be more readily eliminated from the body. This is necessary because when the toxins arrive in the liver they are fat-soluble. In order for them to be eliminated from the body, they need to be converted into water-soluble forms, which is done through oxidation. A special family of enzymes called P-450 makes oxidation possible and thus prepares the fat-soluble toxins for phase 2.

During phase 2, the altered toxins from phase 1 are bound with one of several agents that will make the entire new molecule more water-soluble. Some of these agents include glutathione, glucuronate, and glycine.

Not all toxins go through phase 1, however. Some chemicals are already partially water-soluble, so when they reach the liver they go directly to phase 2, where they are processed and ready for elimination.

Therefore, it is necessary for both phase 1 and phase 2 to be operating optimally for detoxication to be effective. To help ensure that the liver is functioning at full capacity, good nutritional support is key. However, each phase requires some different nutrients (as well as some of the same ones) to complete its job. That's why we conduct a test to identify whether each phase is operating correctly, and if one or both phases are not, we will know which nutrients will help remedy that situation.

Glutathione Levels

Glutathione is an antioxidant that plays a critical role in detoxication in that it conjugates (attaches to) toxic chemicals and helps remove them from the body. Low levels of glutathione can indicate that the body can't adequately perform this essential task, or that it is using all or most of its supply to detoxify the body— suggesting that the body is very toxic. Low levels of glutathione can manifest as fatigue, headache, digestive problems, allergies, and joint pain, as well as multiple sclerosis, lupus, rheumatoid arthritis, and other serious conditions.

❖ OXIDATIVE STRESS PROFILE

When your immune system is impaired and/or you have a deficiency of antioxidants, free radicals can cause a great deal of damage to your body, depleting it of essential nutrients, disrupting communication among cells, and causing various organs and systems to function improperly. This cycle of damage is called oxidative stress. High or low levels of various factors can help doctors determine the degree of oxidative stress your body is experiencing. Because it would not be useful to you for us to list those factors, suffice it to say that there are more than two dozen levels for which we can test.

❖ IMMUNE STUDIES

This category includes a long list of tests whose primary goal is to identify levels of specific substances that are characteristic of different autoimmune processes. Although no single test result can provide a definitive diagnosis, piecing together the results of several carefully chosen tests can reveal a true picture of what is happening at a cellular level in an individual's body. All of the following immune studies are done using a blood sample.

Autoimmune Antibody Tests

Various tests can be used to help diagnose autoimmune disorders. They do this by detecting and measuring the levels of the following autoantibodies.

• **Antinuclear antibodies (ANA),** which may be found in people who have lupus, scleroderma, Sjögren's syndrome, polymyositis, and some types of chronic hepatitis. (ANAs are sometimes also found in the blood of healthy people aged sixty years or older and occasionally in younger people.) Because a positive result on this test can suggest many different conditions, doctors must be careful when they interpret the results. Other tests must also be done to help confirm or rule out their suspicions.

• **Anti-DNA antibody,** which is most typically found in lupus, but occasionally in other autoimmune diseases. Doctors can monitor the anti-DNA antibody levels, which decrease when treatment of lupus is successful. People who have a positive anti-

DNA antibody test usually also have a positive ANA test result. High levels of anti-DNA antibody are associated with glomerulonephritis, an autoimmune disease and a complication of lupus, which is associated with an increased risk of death.

• **Anti–Sm antibody,** an antibody to Sm, a protein found in the nuclei of cells.

• **Anti–smooth muscle antibody (ASMA),** which is often found in people who have autoimmune hepatitis, and frequently in those with ulcerative colitis, rheumatoid arthritis, and polymyositis.

• **Rheumatoid factor (RF),** which is often found in the blood and joint fluids of people who have rheumatoid arthritis. People who have other diseases may also have RF in their blood; thus this test is not specific for rheumatoid arthritis. When RF appears in blood tests of people who are experiencing arthritic pain on both sides of the body, there is a 70 percent chance that they will have joint damage within two years of onset of the disease. High concentrations of RF usually indicate more severe and active disease, more systemic involvement, and a poorer chance for remission.

• **Glomerular basement membrane autoantibody (GBMA),** often found in individuals who have autoimmune kidney disorders, such as glomerulonephritis. The glomerular basement membrane is part of the kidney filtering system; thus damage to this crucial structure can lead to kidney failure. GBMA may also be seen in individuals who have lupus, as kidney problems are common in this disorder.

• **Antineutrophil-cytoplasmic antibody (ANCA)** is an autoantibody that is most common in people who have various forms of vasculitis (inflammation of blood vessels; see chapter 9), as well as rheumatoid arthritis or lupus.

• **Antiphospholipid antibody (APA)** may be seen in people

who have lupus or vasculitis. APAs are believed to cause inflammation and blood vessel damage by attacking platelet membranes or blood vessel walls.

• **Islet cell antibodies (ICAs)** occur in people who have insulin-dependent diabetes (type 1). Approximately 50 to 80 percent of new-onset type 1 diabetics are positive for ICAs, which attack the insulin-producing cells in the pancreas.

All of the above tests infrequently produce false-positive (which indicate antibodies are present when they are not) or false-negative (which indicate antibodies are not present when they are) results. This is one reason why the results of only one test should never be used to make a diagnosis or choose a treatment course.

Complement Levels

Complement is a blood protein that destroys bacteria and also plays a role in inflammation. Abnormal levels of complement are used to detect immunodeficiency, help diagnose autoimmune disorders, and help predict when people with lupus may experience a flare-up. Above-normal levels may indicate the presence of an infection or inflammation, while below-normal levels are often seen in people who have lupus, rheumatoid arthritis, or blood vessel inflammation (vasculitis). A decline in complement levels can signal a flare-up of kidney inflammation in people who have lupus.

Immune Complex Study

Results of this study help doctors diagnose and monitor conditions such as rheumatoid arthritis, lupus, multiple sclerosis, and glomerulonephritis. A blood or synovial (joint) fluid sample is analyzed for the number and type of immune complex molecules present.

Immune complex molecules are formed when antibodies are produced against proteins in the body and these antibodies combine with antigens into a complex, which then circulates throughout the body. These complexes can damage tissues, organs, and joints. For example, the complexes can become trapped in the tubes and blood vessels in the kidney, causing it to leak protein, a condition called glomerulonephritis. In people who have multiple sclerosis, immune complexes are often associated with vision and urinary problems. Immune complexes composed of rheumatoid factors (see "Autoimmune Antibody Tests") can also accumulate in synovial fluid and cause inflammation in the joints as in rheumatoid arthritis.

Cytokine Profile (Inflammatory)

A test for the levels of inflammatory cytokines may be given along with the C-reactive protein test (see below), as both tests reveal markers of systemic inflammation, a sign of lupus, rheumatoid arthritis, CFIDS, and other autoimmune conditions.

TH1-TH2 Cytokine Profile

Cytokines are chemical messengers that control immune responses. This test measures levels of two critical types of cytokines helper T-cell type 1 (TH1) and helper T-cell type 2 (TH2). Low levels of TH1 and high levels of TH2 mean there is an increase in the production of autoantibodies, indicating that an autoimmune process is present. This test may be used for people who appear to have multiple allergies, candidiasis, CFIDS, and other chronic illnesses.

C-Reactive Protein Test

This test detects blood levels of C-reactive protein (CRP), a substance present in the blood of people who have inflammatory disease. It helps diagnose rheumatoid arthritis, which is characterized by high levels of CRP. The C-reactive protein test may be more sensitive than the sedimentation rate in uncovering early- and late-stage infections, but it is more complicated and expensive. If test results show raised levels of CRP and arthritis is suspected, doctors may order that a rheumatoid factor test be done next. If the CRP levels are raised and arthritis is not a symptom, it confirms the presence of systemic inflammation, such as appears in people who have lupus or CFIDS.

Erythrocyte Sedimentation Rate (ESR) Test

This blood test measures how fast red blood cells (erythrocytes) fall to the bottom of a tube that has been filled with a patient's blood. The faster the rate, the greater the extent of inflammation in the body. The problem is, the inflammation may be caused by many autoimmune conditions, including rheumatoid arthritis, lupus, and autoimmune thyroid diseases, as well as nonautoimmune conditions such as anemia, syphilis, cancer, and kidney disease. Therefore, the ESR test is usually used to help identify how serious inflammation is, rather than to identify a disease.

T-Cell Subsets Test

This test detects abnormalities in the levels of immune system cells called lymphocytes. Low levels are associated with immunodeficiency—an inability of the immune system to respond to invading organisms. Specifically, we look at the percentage of two types of T-cells—T4 and T8—which can tell us about various autoimmune processes. Abnormalities of T-cell subsets are seen in some children who have autism. T-cell subset tests are used to help distinguish between inflammatory skin diseases and cancers that can cause rashes.

Immune System Activation of Coagulation Test

The immune system activation of coagulation (ISAC) test measures five substances in blood, and abnormal levels of any two of the five are considered to be positive indications of hypercoagulation. Hypercoagulation (thickened blood) results when too much fibrin (produced by the body to repair wounds and other injuries) is deposited in small blood vessels. Normally, fibrin is made in response to the release of a substance called thrombin. Just one short burst of thrombin is needed to produce a sufficient amount of fibrin. In many people with CFIDS, however, there are abnormal numbers of thrombin bursts, which result in too much fibrin production and ultimately thickened blood. Researchers have found that up to 92 percent of people with CFIDS have hypercoagulation. Symptoms of hypercoagulation include malaise, fatigue, digestive problems, and cognitive problems.

❖ BIOCHEMICAL PROFILE AND CBC

Both of these blood tests provide a wealth of information about the levels of various substances in the body, thus offering clues to existing or potential problems. In that sense they can serve as a foundation for diagnosis and treatment decisions.

- **Biochemical profile** provides levels for more than a dozen elements, including albumin, bilirubin, calcium, chloride, cholesterol, creatinine, glucose, iron, total proteins, and uric acid.
- **Complete blood count** (CBC) is a basic screening test that determines the levels of various blood factors, including hemoglobin, white blood cells, platelets, and others.

❖ NUTRITIONAL STUDIES (IF INDICATED)

Amino Acid Analysis

This analysis is done using blood and urine samples and is used to determine levels of amino acids. Certain enzymes convert or combine with amino acids in the body, resulting in the creation of substances the body uses to function. If certain enzymes are not present, they cannot combine with their designated amino acid, and that particular amino acid continues to accumulate. If amino acid levels are elevated, injury may be indicated; if they are low, rheumatoid arthritis and malnutrition, among other conditions, are suspected.

Organic Acid Analysis

This test is a panel that evaluates various abnormalities, including nutritional deficiencies, antioxidant deficiencies, amino acid and fatty acid abnormalities, overgrowth of yeast and bacteria, and abnormal metabolism of certain neurotransmitters (e.g., serotonin, dopamine), as well as the levels of dozens of compounds. The test is sometimes used in many chronic diseases and in individuals who have symptoms of yeast or bacteria overgrowth.

❖ SENSITIVITY EVALUATION

Allergies and sensitivities to foods and elements in the environment are very common among people who have autoimmune conditions, because the immune system is overactivated, attacking both foreign substances and the body's own cells. Toxins in the body are responsible for these responses.

For example, nearly 90 percent of the food we eat is refined and chemically enhanced. This compares with a mere 25 percent in 1950. Refined foods, such as sugars, coffee, and alcohol, typically pass too quickly into the bloodstream, which may be one reason why so many people have allergic reactions to them. When it comes to chemicals, the average American consumes eight to fifteen pounds of potentially harmful chemicals per year. Some of these chemicals are known to have a negative impact on the digestive system and to contribute to leaky gut syndrome (see chapter 12).

Two basic tests are available to help identify food/inhalant/chemical allergies and sensitivities:

• **Immunoglobulin G radioallergosorbent test.** This blood test, commonly referred to as IgG RAST, measures blood antibodies to food antigens. When the level of antibodies is high, it means the immune system is attacking protein molecules of a specific food in the blood. Food allergies are common among people who have autoimmunity.

• **Skin testing.** Provocation skin testing is the most accurate test for detecting allergies and sensitivities. It is done by injecting a small amount of the suspected allergen under the skin (intradermal). A reddened spot will appear if the individual is allergic or sensitive to the substance. This test works equally well for food and airborne substances.

❖ TESTS FOR SPECIFIC DISEASE GROUPS

Autoimmune Thyroid Disease

A critical test used to diagnose autoimmune thyroid diseases is the comprehensive thyroid autoantibody study, which analyzes the following factors. It is very important to look at the results of all the tests before making a diagnosis.

• **Antithyroglobulin antibodies (ATAs).** Thyroglobulin is a major protein produced by the thyroid gland. It carries the thyroid hormones thyroxine (T4) and T3. ATAs are found in people who have Graves' disease, Hashimoto's thyroiditis, and atrophic thyroiditis. It is less reliable than the anti-TPO test (see below).

• **Antithyroid peroxidase antibodies (anti-TPOs).** Thyroid peroxidase is an enzyme in the thyroid. Antibodies to this enzyme are present in the blood of more than 90 percent of people who have Hashimoto's thyroiditis. This antibody does not cause the disease, but it is a marker for people who have this condition.

• **Thyroid-stimulating hormone (TSH).** The thyroid-stimulating hormone is produced by the pituitary gland. This test measures the amount of TSH in the bloodstream. When TSH levels are below normal, you may be hyper- or hypothyroid; when they are higher, you may be hypothyroid or have a pituitary tumor. A normal reading means you may be euthyroid (normal hormone levels).

• **Thyrotropin-releasing hormone (TRH).** This test is the most sophisticated, as it can identify mild low thyroid, as well as hyperthyroidism. Unlike the TSH test, which measures the amount of thyroid-stimulating hormone normally released by the pituitary, the TRH test measures how much TSH the pituitary stores in reserve. The TRH test is useful for individuals who have symptoms of hypothyroidism or a family history of thyroid disease and a normal TSH level, because it is highly sensitive. However, it is more complicated (three blood draws must be made) and more expensive than the TSH test, so it is usually reserved for cases like those mentioned.

• **Radioactive iodine uptake (RAIU).** This test evaluates thyroid function. An injection of radioactive iodine is given, and the higher the iodine uptake, the more active the thyroid gland. It can be used to confirm a diagnosis of hyperthyroidism, but not hypothyroidism, so it has limited value.

• **Free T4 (FT4).** Most thyroxine (T4) is bound to blood proteins. This test measures the amount of thyroxine that is not, meaning that it is free to enter the cells. The measure of unbound T4 may be helpful, along with the TSH findings, to confirm hypothyroidism.

• **Total serum thyroxine (T4).** This test measures all T4 found that is bound to blood proteins. Thyroxine is the main hormone that controls basal metabolic rate. Abnormally high levels may indicate Graves' disease, hyperthyroidism, acute thyroiditis, or thyroid cancer. Abnormally low levels may indicate hypothyroidism, renal failure, or protein malnutrition. This test is usually done along with TSH and T3.

• **Tri-iodothyronine (T3).** This test measures the amount of T3 in the bloodstream, and is usually done as part of a routine thyroid function evaluation. Abnormally high levels may indicate hyperthyroidism, thyroiditis, or thyroid cancer; abnormally low levels suggest hypothyroidism, chronic illness, or starvation.

Liver

The blood test typically done for liver problems is the autoimmune liver panel, also referred to as the autoimmune liver disease test panel. This blood test measures the levels of albumin (a protein present in the highest concentrations in the blood), gamma globulin, protein, and antibodies in the blood. Any of the following can indicate the presence of chronic active hepatitis:

- Positive test for antinuclear antibodies (ANAs)
- Positive test for anti–smooth muscle antibodies (ASMAs)
- Elevated levels of gamma globulins and low levels of albumin

Ulcerative Colitis and Crohn's Disease

An analysis of a stool sample looks for various bacterial antibodies, including those for bacterial endotoxins, bacterial exotoxins, *C. difficile,* klebsiella, and *Yersinia.* So far, no autoantibodies have definitively been associated with ulcerative colitis and Crohn's disease.

Neurological Disorders

Autoantibodies to the following factors are typically found in people whose autoimmune process affects their nervous system. This includes people who have multiple sclerosis, myasthenia gravis, and other demyelinating conditions, as well as autism.

Several of these factors are mentioned in this book; the others are those I also check for on a patient-by-patient basis.

- Myelin basic protein: a brain protein of the myelin sheath, which protects the nerve cells and is essential for higher brain function.
- Myelin oligodendrocytes: myelin is produced by nervous system cells called oligodendrocytes; thus autoantibodies against these cells further myelin damage.
- Ganglioside: a substance found in the highest concentrations in nerve cell membranes. It has an important role in cell growth, development, and repair.
- Tubulin: a key protein in cell division and the movement of materials inside cells.
- Cerebellar (Purkinje): nerve cells in the brain (cerebellum, the part of the brain responsible for coordination), which play a key role in message transmission.

Part II

❖

COMMON AUTOIMMUNE DISEASES

Chapter 3

Autism

Many readers may be surprised to find autism in a book about autoimmune disorders. One reason is that when most people think of an autoimmune disorder, they think about physical medical problems, such as muscle pain, fatigue, inflammation, gastrointestinal problems, and the like. Autism, however, is generally viewed as a psychological and behavioral disorder, and in fact at one time it was referred to as childhood schizophrenia. True, people who have autism do display various unusual behaviors and psychological responses. Yet what is at the root of those behaviors and responses? It is my sincere belief, and there is overwhelming evidence, that autism is associated with heavy metal and chemical toxicity, and that those environmental poisons trigger autoimmunity.

In this chapter we will explore those roots and why autism has become an epidemic in this country. We will also discuss how I and some other physicians are using innovative approaches to treat the rapidly growing number of children who are diagnosed with this disorder. It is our hope that we can shed some light and hope for those parents who have a child diagnosed with autism, and for those individuals who are not yet parents but who want to help prevent the disorder from developing in their yet-unborn children. Therefore this chapter is dedicated to the millions of children and their family members who are affected by and live with autism.

❖ AUTISM YESTERDAY AND TODAY

From 1800 to 1943, the condition known today as autism—or more accurately, autistic spectrum disorder, because it has so many facets—was viewed as a type of schizophrenia. It was a rare disease, and didn't attract a significant amount of attention until 1943, when Leo Kanner, a child psychiatrist, described a behavioral disorder in which children had repetitive behaviors, were socially withdrawn, and lacked meaningful speech, facial expression, and eye contact. He labeled the syndrome early infantile autism (autism, from the Greek word *autos,* meaning "self").

At the time, autism was thought to be purely a behavioral disorder. Since then, however, researchers have learned that it is a multifaceted condition that involves not only the brain but also the immune system and the gastrointestinal tract. With this discovery, the term "autistic spectrum disorder" was introduced.

Autism was rare before Kanner's time and remained relatively uncommon for several decades. In the 1960s, the incidence of autism was 1 child out of every 2,000. By the year 2000 that number had ballooned to 1 to 2 in 500, and in some pockets of the United States, autism has been reported to be as common as 1 in 132 children. Clearly, autism is an epidemic.

❖ IS AUTISM AN AUTOIMMUNE DISORDER?

I first became interested in a possible connection between environmental toxins, autoimmunity, and autism in 1994 when an autistic patient was brought to my Center for evaluation. My subsequent intense investigation and research uncovered much convincing evidence that such a link exists. For example:

• In 1975, the National Institutes of Health did a study in which they followed 55,908 pregnancies and subsequent births. Fourteen of the children had infantile autism. Although this was a low number, the fact that there was a higher incidence of the mother's job involving chemicals in these 14 children was clear.

• In 1976, a study conducted at the Children's Brain Research Clinic in Washington, D.C., found that among 78 children with autism, the parents' exposure to environmental chemicals *before conception* was a statistically significant factor in 20 families. A second similar study done in 1981 also saw a statistically significant increase in the number of cases of autism.

• In 1977, a study of 12 children with autism showed that all 12 had a deficiency of T-cells. This deficiency is also seen in people who have burdens of chemicals and heavy metals.

• In 1997, researchers found that children with autism have a greater frequency of antibodies to certain brain cells than do healthy children, pointing to autoimmunity and a role for these antibodies in disrupting language and social development.

• In England, Dr. Waring found that more than 90 percent of autistic children have a deficiency of a specific enzyme (phenosulfotransferase), a deficiency that prevents the liver from properly detoxifying foreign chemicals.

• Numerous other studies have shown that a significant number of autistic children have immune system activities characteristic of autoimmunity, including reduced natural killer cell activity, abnormal T-cell activity, and an altered ratio of helper T-cells to T-suppressor cells (see chapter 1).

Some very convincing evidence comes from Vijendra K. Singh, Ph.D., of Utah State University and the Autism Auto-immunity Project. Dr. Singh has intensively studied autism and autoimmunity for nearly twenty years and states that "I firmly believe that up to eighty percent (and possibly all) cases of autism are caused by an abnormal immune reaction, commonly known as autoimmunity." His statement is based on data from approximately four hundred cases (autism and controls), in which he found that up to 80 percent of autistic children have autoantibodies to certain brain structures, especially the myelin basic protein found in the myelin sheath, a coating that protects nerve fibers. While these autoantibodies are found in 65 to 85 percent of children who have autism, they are rarely seen (0 to 5 percent) in healthy children.

❖ CAUSES, TRIGGERS, AND RISK FACTORS

Most experts agree that autism is a complex disorder, and that many factors are involved. I believe those factors fall into two main categories—genetics and environmental toxins—and that these two elements together are at the root of autism.

Genetics and Environmental Toxins

Little is known about the genetics of autism. More males than females have autism, which leads researchers to believe that the condition may be associated with a nonworking gene on the X (male) chromosome. However, the presence of this gene is not believed to be responsible for the majority of cases. Some studies suggest that families that have one child with autism have an increased risk of 4 percent that another child will also have the disorder.

My experience and research have shown me that the genetics of autism concerns the liver and possibly its inability to effectively or efficiently detoxify chemicals. The developing fetus gets the toxins from its mother, who has ingested them in food and from her environment. Excessive amounts of heavy metals and chemicals, along with the infant's inability to deal with them, leads to free-radical production, which damages the brain and other organs.

This idea is supported by one of my own studies from 1998. In that study, we evaluated 20 autistic children and found that 19 had abnormal toxic chemical blood levels, and all had abnormal immune system activity, disrupted liver detoxication, and nutritional deficiencies. These results indicate that autistic spectrum disorder probably involves damage in the brain caused by environmental chemicals. In addition, the presence of nutritional deficiencies makes it nearly impossible for the body to effectively eliminate the toxins from the body.

There is no question in my mind that heavy metals and chemicals are at the roots of most cases of autism. When we look at the work of Dr. Singh, we see that about 80 percent of autistic children have autoantibodies, especially to myelin basic protein, which affects the nervous system. (My own study shows about 50 percent. The truth may lie somewhere in between. But this we know: the number is significant.)

The production of these autoantibodies is seen again and again in people with autoimmunity who are toxic for heavy metals and chemicals. In children with autism, these toxins damage not only the myelin sheaths but also nerve structures and possibly even enzyme systems within the cells, all of which factors work together to cause the unusual behaviors and psychological problems experienced by these children.

Vaccinations and Toxins

Some researchers are pointing to a relationship between childhood vaccinations and the development of autism. Clearly, not every child who gets vaccinations develops the disorder, yet there have been enough cases to cause some concern. I believe that concern can be linked to the fact that most childhood vaccines, up until very recently, contained mercury. Now all childhood vaccines have at least one mercury-free version, and I urge parents to ask for those versions if they choose to vaccinate their children. Injecting mercury into children, especially infants whose immune systems are still underdeveloped (hepatitis B shots are typically given at birth, before the immune system has developed), can be an assault to the immune system.

❖ SIGNS AND SYMPTOMS

Children with autism can display a wide range of signs and symptoms. Here are just a few:

- Abnormal movements, such as arm-flapping, spinning, rocking, moving in circles, difficulties crawling
- Sensory abnormalities, such as oversensitivity to sound, aversion to being touched
- Speech and hearing problems, such as delay or failure to develop speech, mild to severe hearing loss, problems with word use
- Visual problems, such as poor eye contact (will not meet the eyes of other people), blurred vision

- Cognitive problems, such as poor concentration, difficulty comprehending words or following multiple commands
- Unusual behaviors, such as head-banging, staring, social isolation
- Physical problems, such as poor muscle strength (especially in the upper body), abnormal sweating, diarrhea, constipation, seizures, tendency to have allergies and asthma, likely to have a family history of autoimmune disorders

Many people recognize these characteristics of autism, but what most people don't know is that all of them are also symptoms of mercury poisoning and other toxic problems. This fact, to me, seems like clear evidence that autism may have roots in heavy metal and chemical toxicity.

❖ DIAGNOSIS AND TREATMENT OF AUTISM: CONVENTIONAL APPROACH

Because there are no medical tests that can be used to diagnose autism, doctors must make their diagnosis based on their observations of the individual's behavior, development skills, and communication skills. (Some medical tests may be used, however, to rule out other disorders that have some symptoms similar to those seen in autism.) When we say "doctors," we mean a medical team, because it takes experts in several areas to make an accurate diagnosis of autism. Such a team may include a child and adolescent psychiatrist, psychologist, developmental pediatrician, speech/language therapist, neurologist, learning disorder specialist, and any other professionals who are knowledgeable about autism.

These professionals may use terms such as "autistic-like," "high-functioning autism," and "low-functioning autism" when making their diagnosis. That's because autism is a spectrum disorder, with symptoms and characteristics that can range from mild to severe, and appear in many different combinations, from child to child.

Diagnosing Autism

After experts have observed an individual and done tests to rule out other conditions (e.g., mental retardation, deafness), a diagnosis of autism is made only if the following symptoms are clear:

- repetitive activities, behaviors, and interests
- underdeveloped communication skills
- limited or poor ability to form social relationships

These symptoms can be of varying intensity, but according to diagnostic criteria, they must appear by the time the child is three years old.

Treating Autism

Because autism is a complex disorder, treatment also requires a multifaceted approach. Conventional medicine uses a limited approach, utilizing speech and occupational therapy, along with drugs, when necessary, to treat symptoms. Speech and language therapy is critical for autistic children because it helps them with communication and social development. Drug therapy, including antidepressants, is rarely helpful in treating autism. However, it is not unusual for doctors to treat symptoms with drugs. Hyperactive children, for example, may be given Ritalin, while those who have trouble sleeping may be given clonidine. All of these approaches are usually covered by insurance.

Some individuals are willing and/or have the financial means to try other methods considered to be alternative or nonconventional. Research shows that people who are autistic respond best when they are presented with highly structured programs that may include (but are not limited to) any of the following (which generally are not covered by insurance):

• Applied behavior analysis (ABA). This is a highly effective and intensive approach that is based on positive reinforcement. In most cases, it involves one-on-one sessions with the child for thirty to forty hours per week for a year or more.

• Auditory integration training. This method helps modulate and control the volume of sound frequencies in individuals who are hypersensitive to sound. Auditory integration training can help reduce hypersensitivity, improve language discrimination and verbalization, and reduce irritability.

• Dietary therapy. Elimination of foods that contain the proteins gluten (from wheat) and casein (from dairy) has been successful in some cases. The effectiveness of this approach may be associated with the fact that some people with autism are not able to break down certain proteins.

• Music or art therapy. These therapies allow children to express themselves in nonverbal ways.

• Sensory integration. This is an approach that helps individuals who misinterpret sensations from their environment, which causes them to have problems with information processing and behavior. Sensory integration involves three areas—touch, balance, and awareness of body position and motor abilities—and helps people interpret external stimuli so they can respond appropriately.

• Alternative nutrition therapies, including the use of magnesium, vitamin B_6, dimethyl-glycine (DMG, an amino acid compound), and certain amino acids, have been useful in some patients, but they should be used only under a doctor's strict supervision.

The problem with all of these therapies—conventional and alternative—is that they don't address the cause of the behavior problems. They need to be done in combination with a program that eliminates heavy metals and chemicals from the body.

❖ EVALUATION AND TREATMENT OF AUTISM: MY APPROACH

Given that autism is such a complex, multifaceted phenomenon, I believe it is necessary to evaluate each patient using a comprehensive analysis that allows me to get a complete picture of the causes and triggers of the disorder. That analysis necessarily includes information about heavy metal and chemical exposures and many other characteristics.

Evaluation

Because we are dealing with young children, my evaluation process involves asking parents a lot of questions. I collect historical information, ranging from the time of conception to the present, as well as information about the lives of the parents before conception. Of particular interest are environmental influences (e.g., exposure to toxins at home or at work), nutritional factors, and dental history, especially of the mother. The child is given a complete physical examination, and an analysis of laboratory specimens (urine, blood, stool) is done to help determine the origins of the illness and any accompanying symptoms.

At the Edelson Center, the typical testing process for autistic children is very extensive and involves various tests in each of the following categories: immunological, toxicological, nutritional/ biochemical, gastrointestinal, infectious, autoimmune, renal function, and liver detoxication. Rather than explain these tests, I refer you to my book *Conquering Autism: Reclaiming Your Child through Natural Therapies* for details on autism. To give you an example of the patients whom I see and treat, let's look at Brittany's story.

Evaluating Brittany

Two weary adults with an expressionless five-year-old girl in tow greeted me at the Center one day in 1998. Brittany had been diagnosed with autism at age two and a half. She was proving to be a handful for her parents, who reported the following characteristics: severe temper tantrums, a fascination with mechanical objects, severely limited diet, often violent reaction to being touched, poor motor skills, erratic sleep behavior, extreme fear of simple expectations (such as going to the store) but no fear of dangerous or life-threatening situations, social detachment, and inappropriate play with toys and other objects. She also suffered with frequent bouts of diarrhea and stomach upset.

Brittany's parents had been relentless in their search for help; they had already consulted more than a dozen pediatricians and environmental medical doctors, more than a dozen psychologists and behaviorists, and more than another dozen alternative practitioners, occupational therapists, and speech therapists. Even with all that, they had seen barely any improvement.

When I questioned the parents about environmental exposures, I learned that Karyn, the mother, had had dental work during her first trimester, including an amalgam (mercury) filling. She also had six other fillings already in her mouth from her teenage years. Tim, her husband, had been a smoker until Brittany was born, when he quit. However, Karyn had been exposed to secondhand smoke before and during her entire pregnancy.

Brittany had received all her routine vaccinations, including hepatitis B (which contained mercury) one day after her birth. Karyn was unsure which of the other vaccines contained mercury, but we assumed that at least the two subsequent hepatitis B vaccines contained the toxin.

When I tested Brittany for heavy metals and chemical toxicity, I found very high levels of mercury and high levels of various chemicals. She also showed deficiencies of several B vitamins as well as zinc, selenium, and vitamin A; malabsorption (seen on the CDSA); leaky gut syndrome; an overgrowth of candida; and food allergies to wheat and dairy.

Treatment

Based on the findings from her evaluation, I recommended the following treatment program for Brittany.

• Nutritional therapy. Brittany was given supplements not only to address the deficiencies that were revealed on her tests but also to maintain healthy levels of nutrients lost during biodetoxification. She received a special formulation of vitamins, minerals, amino acids, and enzymes for her specific needs.

• Immunotherapy. We started Brittany on a program of EPD (enzyme potentiated desensitization) to eliminate her food allergies.

• Environmental controls. Brittany's parents were told to institute environmental controls in their home, including the use of water filters and HEPA (high-efficiency particulate arresting) air filters, avoidance of household and garden chemicals, elimination of foods containing food additives, and introduction of organic foods.

• Chelation. A program of oral DMSA and intravenous DMPS. The DMSA crosses the blood-brain barrier and can remove heavy metals from the brain.

• High-temperature sauna therapy. Brittany went through the month-long biodetoxification program, which included high-temperature therapy. Brittany's parents took turns staying in the sauna with their daughter, and she did remarkably well with the therapy.

• Intravenous gamma globulin. This treatment can suppress the production of autoantibodies, and has proved helpful in the treatment of autism. Brittany received treatment for six months.

• Ozone therapy. To eliminate Brittany's candida infection, we used autohemotherapy, which, while it does not destroy candida directly, improves immune system function, which in turn supports the destruction of infectious organisms.

• Pancreatic enzymes. Daily supplementation with pancreatic enzymes was initiated to address maldigestion.

I also recommended that Brittany begin applied behavioral analysis, a form of behavioral therapy that has proved successful in helping many autistic children. She had been seeing a speech/language therapist at the time she first came to see me, and she continued with that therapy. Within a few months, Brittany was showing much improvement in speech, eye contact, socialization, and temperament. Her frequent severe temper tantrums had dwindled to periodic, milder events. Her sleep improved, allowing her parents to get much-needed sleep themselves. After a year of treatment, Brittany's heavy metal and chemical toxicity burden had been reduced to within safe limits. And the changes in her temperament and behavior were dramatic. Karyn and Tim said Brittany was a completely different child. She allowed her parents to hold her, her language skills had improved dramatically, and she interacted with other children. Today Brittany is a bright, active child who attends mainstream classes in public school.

❖ CLOSING THOUGHTS ON AUTISM

Autism is a devastating condition that must, in my opinion, be addressed on two fronts. One is aggressive treatment that includes attention to the environmental and immunological aspects of the syndrome—namely, biodetoxification and immunotherapy. The longer we wait to treat autistic children in this manner, the greater the possibility that we will not be able to reverse the process that is damaging the nervous system.

The other front is prevention. I believe that intensive preconceptual counseling is critical if we are to stop this epidemic. Why? In 1999, researchers found a strong relationship between people who had a family history of autoimmune disorders and autism. In their study, individuals who had two or more family members with an autoimmune condition were twice as likely to have autism. When at least three family members had an autoimmune condition, the risk increased to 5.5 times. If the child's mother had an autoimmune disorder, the risk increased to 8.8 times.

Both parents need to be free of toxicity before they conceive. They both need to understand how to prevent environmental toxins from affecting them and their unborn child and, once the child is born, how to continue to live in a relatively toxin-free environment (see chapter 11). Living toxin-free extends to the use of childhood vaccinations. Parents need to be informed about the benefits and risks of any vaccination and know that they have a legal right to refuse any one or more of them. I believe that if immunizations are given at all, they should be administered after a child is at least one year old, when his or her immune system has developed to a point where it can better handle the assault.

We will not wipe out autism overnight. But we can take giant steps in the right direction if we are willing to broaden our view of what is at the root of autism and are willing to act responsibly and not expose our unborn children to a toxic environment.

❖ WHAT YOU CAN DO NOW

If your child has autism:

• Find a doctor who performs the tests and uses the treatments discussed in this chapter (see chapter 2).

• Become familiar with the pros and cons of childhood vaccinations and learn about your right to refuse to vaccinate your child. To get the information relevant to your state, contact your state's department of public health and ask that your state's laws on vaccinations be sent to you.

• Make your home environment as toxin-free as possible (see chapter 11 for specific suggestions). I recommend installation of HEPA filters and water filters, and avoidance of all pesticides, insecticides, herbicides, and household cleaning chemicals.

• Switch to a whole foods, organic diet that includes lots of fruits and vegetables and whole grains. You want to avoid hormones, steroids, and food additives, preservatives, and colorings. This way of eating is healthy for the entire family, and if everyone eats the same way, the autistic child will not feel different or alienated.

• Have your child tested for food allergies.

• Read more about the autism/environmental metal link and what you can do in *Conquering Autism: Reclaiming Your Child through Natural Therapies.*

Chapter 4

Lupus

In 1953, when Henrietta Aladjen was diagnosed with lupus, she was told she had a rare disease that mostly affected people with blond hair and blue eyes. Henrietta, a native of Hungary, fit that physical profile. She was also told that the disease was usually fatal.

Well, we didn't know much about lupus back then. And although there is much about lupus we still do not understand, we do know that it is an autoimmune disease that affects blacks, Latinos, Asians, and Native Americans more than it does whites (there goes the blond/blue eyes theory) and that it is not invariably fatal. We also know that it affects women about nine times as often as men, that it is a complex, chronic disease that affects at least 1.5 million Americans, and that it continues to baffle medical science. As for Henrietta, she went on to found the Lupus Foundation of America, and she was honored by President Ronald Reagan in 1985 for her work in advancing understanding of the disease.

❖ WHAT IS LUPUS?

Why the word "lupus," which is Latin for "wolf," was chosen to describe this disease is a mystery. The word "lupus" is usually used to refer to the most common form of the disease—systemic lupus erythematosus, or SLE. SLE is an autoimmune disorder that causes inflammation in various organ systems in the body, hence the description "systemic." The systems are damaged because the body produces antibodies that react with the cells in these systems, resulting in symptoms such as rash (skin), arthritis (joints), nephritis (kidney inflammation), myocardial dysfunction and various cardiac abnormalities (heart), and anemia (blood). "Erythematosus" means "red," which describes the rash that affects many people who have SLE.

About 90 percent of people with SLE are young women aged fifteen to forty-five. In the United States, black women get the disease three times more often than do white women—1 in every 250 black women has the disease—and Asians, Native Americans, and Latinos get it about twice as often as women of European descent. Symptoms, including fatigue, arthritis, rash, and others (see "Signs and Symptoms," below) typically come and go at irregular intervals and can range from mild to severe.

❖ WHY LUPUS IS AN AUTOIMMUNE DISEASE

The autoimmune process that occurs in what is commonly diagnosed as lupus typically involves three types of immune system cells: macrophages, B-cells, and helper T-cells. The macrophages encounter the foreign substance, or antigen, whether it be a virus, a chemical compound, mercury, or other environmental factor (see "Causes, Triggers, and Risk Factors," below). The macrophages then display a fragment of the antigen on their surface,

and the helper T-cells recognize the antigen. The T-cells then produce chemicals called lymphokines, which stimulate the B-cells
to attack the antigens. The process is now in full swing as free radicals are mass-produced, and various cells and organ systems become inflamed and damaged. Most of the criteria for lupus are
definite autoimmune responses (see "The Criteria for SLE,"
below).

❖ FORMS OF LUPUS

In addition to SLE, there are two other forms of lupus that are
much less common: discoid lupus, which affects the skin only;
and drug-induced lupus. Symptoms of discoid lupus, also known
as cutaneous lupus, include various types of rash, photosensitivity (when exposure to sunlight triggers a rash), and ulcers on the
inside of the mouth or nose. About 10 percent of people with discoid lupus develop SLE, but so far no one is able to predict which
individuals will get the systemic disease. Discoid lupus affects
more men than does SLE.

Drug-induced lupus develops in more men than women because most of the drugs that cause this disorder are taken more
often by men. The two most common lupus-inducing drugs are
procainamide, which is used to treat heart irregularities, and
hydralazine, which is used to control high blood pressure. Symptoms of this form of lupus usually disappear within weeks to
months after individuals stop taking the drug.

❖ CAUSES, TRIGGERS, AND RISK FACTORS

Medical researchers are not certain about the origins of SLE, but
most agree that it involves a complex number of factors working
together. The disease occurs when a specific set of genes predis-

posed to the disease are triggered by a combination of factors, all of which we discuss below.

Genetics

The importance of the inherited predisposition for lupus probably differs among individuals who have the disorder, with environmental triggers like viruses, drugs, or heavy metals having a bigger influence on some people, while others may have a stronger genetic predisposition with environmental factors playing a lesser role. In either case, it is generally believed that a combination of genetics and environmental factors cause lupus.

One piece of evidence supporting a genetic tendency for lupus came in February 1997, when researchers at the University of California at Los Angeles said they had found a gene that makes people vulnerable to lupus. Another piece surfaced in September 2001, when scientists at the University of Colorado Health Center announced they had identified a gene that increases the risk of developing lupus.

Researchers believe that more than one gene determines whether a person will get the disease, and that these genes interact with environmental triggers to cause the disease. Not everyone who has the lupus gene gets the disease, however. That appears to depend on individuals being exposed to the right triggers.

In early 2001, Jamey Marth, M.D., and his fellow researchers at the University of California at San Diego announced that they had identified a genetic defect in mice that triggers a disease process that is very similar to lupus in humans. Although we are not mice, scientists believe this finding is a significant clue to how lupus and other autoimmune conditions involve abnormalities in the way the body makes carbohydrates. They believe the defect may change carbohydrates that reside on the cells' surface enough so that the immune system identifies them as invaders and attacks them.

For now this is speculation. But several things make this finding interesting. One is that earlier studies have found that some patients with other autoimmune disorders also process carbohydrates in an unusual way. This parallel supports the idea that most autoimmune conditions have similar origins. Also of interest, says Marth, is that "what we put into the body," including food and substances that enter involuntarily, such as air pollutants, second-hand smoke, pesticide residue, and household chemicals, can change cell-surface carbohydrates. Thus environmental toxins may be the triggering mechanism in lupus.

Environmental Factors

Lupus is one autoimmune disorder in which scientists have evidence that environmental factors trigger the disease. One bit of evidence is the fact that one form of lupus is drug-induced. Once individuals stop taking the culprit drug and it is cleared out of their system, lupus symptoms go away.

Yet in most cases the triggering mechanisms appear to be things other than drugs. In all cases of lupus that I see, elevated levels of heavy metals, chemicals, or both are involved. Exposure to ultraviolet light triggers symptoms in about one-third of patients. Infections (cold, flu, bronchitis, and so on), emotional stress, and physical trauma can also trigger the disease.

Hormonal factors may explain why lupus occurs more frequently in women than in men. In particular, estrogen may be partly responsible for the increase in disease symptoms that often occurs in women before their menstrual periods and during pregnancy. The exact role of hormones, however, has not yet been identified.

Enzyme Deficiency

In June 2000, the journal *Nature Genetics* reported that scientists had found direct evidence that a deficiency in an enzyme called Dnase-1 leads to SLE. Dnase-1's task is to break down DNA strands after cells have died to make cleanup and their elimination from the body easier. The study showed that, in mice at least, when this breakdown process is disturbed, the body initiates an autoimmune response. The researchers also looked at ten patients with SLE and kidney disease and found that four of them had significantly reduced Dnase-1 activity.

Although these results are preliminary, they suggest that in the near future, doctors may test for a Dnase-1 deficiency to help identify people who are at risk of developing the disease.

Family History

Family history also plays a role in the development of lupus. Ten percent of people with lupus have a parent or sibling who has or who will develop the disease, and about 5 percent of the children born to women with lupus will develop the condition.

❖ SIGNS AND SYMPTOMS

"I feel as if I'm on a roller-coaster," says Samantha, a thirty-eight-year-old mother of two. "Most of the time I'm tired, but when my symptoms flare up, I am so fatigued I can't get out of bed in the morning. All my joints ache, and I get a rash on my face and arms. These symptoms will last for weeks, sometimes a month or

more, and then go away. I never know when they're going to
come back. And when they do, I may have a new symptom to
contend with. I live in fear all the time—afraid that next time my
symptoms come back I'll be too sick to take care of my kids."

Samantha's situation is not unusual. People with lupus can
experience many different symptoms that can come and go unexpectedly. When one symptom goes away, patients don't know if
they will get it again or if another one will take its place, when it
will come, or how serious it will be.

Lupus is a disease of uncertainty. It can affect virtually every
organ and organ system in the body at any given time. Some of
the most common symptoms patients experience, and the percentage who experience them, include:

Achy joints (arthralgia): 95%
Fever greater than 100°F: 90%
Arthritis (swollen joints): 90%
Prolonged or severe fatigue: 81%
Myocardial dysfunction: up to 78%
Rash: 74%
Anemia: 71%
Cardiac abnormalities: up to 55%
Kidney involvement (inflammation): 50%
Butterfly rash: 42%
Photosensitivity: 30%
Hair loss: 27%
Abnormal blood clotting: 20%
Raynaud's disease (cold extremities): 17%
Seizures: 15%
Migraine: 10 to 37%

Depression: The "Other" Symptom of Lupus

"When I first got the diagnosis of lupus, I felt relieved that someone had finally validated my illness," says Trudi, a forty-year-old bookkeeper. "But then all I could think about was that I had heard lupus was fatal. Even when my doctor tried to reassure me that it wasn't necessarily true, I wasn't convinced. I became very depressed."

Depression is very common among people who have lupus. One reason is that the multiple symptoms leave many people unable to continue with their normal lifestyle, including work, school, and social activities. For people who are in a sexual relationship, difficulties with sex can be a problem because of the pain and fatigue. Another reason is that the facial rash affects appearance. Especially for young women, this can be a great source of embarrassment. And then there are the side effects of treatment: people who use steroids (see "Treatment") usually experience weight gain, puffy cheeks, and stretch marks, which further lower self-esteem.

Support groups can offer significant help for anyone who has lupus, regardless of the treatment path—conventional or alternative—they choose. Sharing with others who have the condition can provide moral and spiritual strength, validation of feelings, and practical tips on how to cope with symptoms, family, friends, work, and emotional and social issues.

❖ DIAGNOSIS AND TREATMENT OF LUPUS: CONVENTIONAL APPROACH

Over the course of three years, Diane consulted four doctors before she got a diagnosis of lupus. Jerry wasn't so lucky. He saw six doctors, most of whom said, "Your symptoms are all in your head," before he received a diagnosis. His search took nearly five years. During all the years they searched for answers, Diane and Jerry felt frustration, anger, fear, and doubt. Many times they felt like they would never find someone to help them. But at the same time they knew that the symptoms they were experiencing were real, and that they were ruining their lives.

What's the Problem?

Diane and Jerry are not alone. People who have symptoms of lupus and similar disorders often find it difficult to find a healthcare professional who can validate their experiences. What's the problem? Lupus is a difficult condition to diagnose because:

- It is a multisystem disease, so in order for an individual to meet the required criteria for diagnosis (see "The Criteria for SLE"), it is necessary for symptoms to be present in different parts of the body and for tests to back up their presence.
- SLE mimics many other diseases and conditions, which means that to get a diagnosis, doctors must do tests that eliminate other conditions.
- SLE tends to develop slowly over months or even years, and symptoms come and go, so it can take time for enough symptoms to present themselves and for a diagnosis to be made.
- There is no single diagnostic test for lupus, so several tests may need to be given.

If you refer to chapter 10 on chronic fatigue and immune dysfunction syndrome, you will notice that this condition shares many of the same characteristics as lupus. This is no coincidence: as I've mentioned, most autoimmune conditions share many characteristics, and that's because what ties them together is the autoimmune process that's occurring at the cellular level. That's the level at which we must work to stop autoimmunity and return the body to health.

The Criteria for SLE

The American College of Rheumatology developed a list of criteria for diagnosing SLE. People need to meet at least four of these criteria before a diagnosis of lupus can be made.

• Malar rash: a persistent flat or raised rash that appears on the cheeks and bridge of the nose. The rash may burn or itch or be hot to the touch. About half of all lupus patients experience malar rash. Biopsies of these rashes reveal antibodies and inflammation of the blood vessels, which confirms the presence of autoimmunity.

• Discoid rash: raised red patches with scaling and scarring. This affects about 25 percent of patients. The presence of inflamed cells validates an autoimmune response.

• Photosensitivity: symptoms that develop as a reaction to sunlight or other forms of light (i.e., fluorescent and halogen light). Light exposure may provoke rash, fever, joint pain, heart palpitations, fatigue, and even kidney disease.

• Oral ulcers (aphthous ulcers): painless lesions in the mouth that resemble cold sores. Affect about 40 percent of patients.

• Arthritis: swelling and tenderness in joints in the arms, legs, feet, and hands. Most lupus patients have some form of arthritis.

• Serositis: inflammation of the covering of the lung, abdominal cavity, or heart. About half of all lupus patients have this symptom.

• Kidney problems: most lupus patients have some type of kidney difficulty, which can range from mild (e.g., leaking protein into the urine) to severe (failure of the kidney to remove toxins from the blood). About half of lupus patients with kidney involvement experience permanent kidney damage.

• Neurological problems: a wide range of central nervous system (CNS) problems are possible, including seizures, memory problems, confusion, severe depression, and psychosis. About 50 percent of patients have some kind of CNS difficulty.

• Blood abnormalities: four different blood disorders are commonly found in people with lupus. These are caused by auto-antibodies that attack specific blood cells: (1) hemolytic anemia, where people produce antibodies to their own red blood cells; (2) leukopenia, where the white blood cell level is low, indicating an active case of lupus; (3) thrombocytopenia, where autoantibodies destroy the platelets, which can cause bleeding; and (4) lymphocytopenia, low lymphocyte levels, which hinders the body's ability to fight infection.

• Immunological problems: five blood abnormalities that indicate lupus, including the presence of anti-DNA, anti-Sm and antinuclear (ANA) antibodies, the presence of the lupus erythematosus (LE) cell (not reliable; I personally do not use it), and a false-positive test result for syphilis. The LE cell is also often found in patients who have other autoimmune diseases, such as rheumatoid arthritis, Sjögren's syndrome, and scleroderma. The fact that it is found in other autoimmune disorders supports the idea that autoimmune conditions have many similarities and can therefore be treated in a similar fashion, regardless of the diagnosis.

Testing for SLE

The criteria for diagnosing SLE are very specific about which blood and immunological problems are required; thus doctors have a select list of tests that they usually conduct. Here are the ones you can likely expect if you visit a conventional physician.

• ANA (antinuclear antibody) test. Often referred to as a "lupus test." Although 95 percent of people with SLE have positive ANA test results, most people who have positive ANA do not have lupus. A positive result can also be found in individuals who have conditions such as rheumatoid arthritis, Sjögren's syndrome, mononucleosis, malaria, autoimmune liver disease, autoimmune thyroid disease, scleroderma, or subacute bacterial endocarditis (inflammation of the lining of the heart cavity). People who have many symptoms of SLE but have a negative ANA test generally are not diagnosed with lupus, but that does not mean they do not have autoimmunity.

• Anti-DNA antibody test. Anti-DNA antibodies are usually seen along with a positive ANA. A definite positive result on this test, along with symptoms of lupus, nearly always means the individual has lupus. Because this test is rarely positive in other illnesses, it is a good predictor of lupus.

• Anti-Sm antibody test. Checks for antibodies against Sm, a ribonucleoprotein found in the nuclei of cells. This test is highly specific for SLE, and these antibodies are rarely found in patients with other rheumatic diseases, such as rheumatoid arthritis. However, only 30 percent of patients with SLE have a positive result on their anti-Sm test.

• LE cell test. Lupus erythematosus cells are seen in 40 to 50 percent of people who have lupus. Unfortunately, this test can also be positive in up to 20 percent of patients who have rheumatoid arthritis, and in a smaller percentage of people with other autoimmune conditions, such as scleroderma and Sjögren's syndrome.

• Complement levels. This blood test measures the total level of complement, a group of proteins that can occur in immune system reactions. If the total complement level is low, or if specific complements (C3 and C4) are low and the patient also has a positive ANA test result, a diagnosis of lupus is likely.

A major problem with depending on these tests to diagnose lupus is that they are not effective in the early stages of the disease. Therefore, doctors who practice conventional medicine don't "see" anything wrong, don't recognize that an autoimmune process is at the root of the symptoms, and send the patient home. Clinical molecular physicians like myself explore deeper—using heavy metal testing, nutritional testing, and so on—to identify what's happening at a cellular level, and can thus begin appropriate treatment to stop the autoimmune process.

Treatment

The purpose of conventional treatment is to minimize symptoms, reduce inflammation, help maintain normal bodily functioning, and prevent flare-ups. Most doctors prescribe drugs to achieve these goals, choosing the drugs based on the organ systems affected and the severity of the symptoms.

Before Brenda, a thirty-nine-year-old paralegal with two children, came to my clinic, she had been diagnosed with lupus for four years. Except for two general recommendations by her doctor—to protect herself from the sun because she was photosensitive and to avoid temperature extremes because of Raynaud's phenomenon—she was trying to manage her symptoms with drugs.

"Juggling all the drugs and dealing with the side effects became a nightmare," said Brenda. "My symptoms would keep changing—sometimes they were bad, sometimes not so bad—and then I wouldn't know which were worse, the symptoms or the side effects of the drugs. I was so frustrated with the doctors, the drugs, and myself, and I knew I had to find a better way to deal with this disease."

Brenda's frustration is shared by many lupus patients who are taking multiple numbers of drugs for relief. Here are the main medications often prescribed by doctors, their effectiveness, and side effects.

Corticosteroids

Corticosteroids, or steroids, are considered the backbone of lupus treatment, because of their ability to reduce inflammation and suppress the activity of the immune system. These hormones are available in several forms, including creams (for rashes and oral ulcers), injections (for arthritis pain), and pills. The most commonly prescribed steroid is prednisone; prednisolone and triamcinolone are popular as well. Although steroids are effective, people who take them for a month or longer can expect adverse reactions, including:

- Increased appetite, which can result in weight gain
- Raised blood sugar levels
- Increased risk of developing infection because they suppress the immune system
- "Moon face," caused by a redistribution of fat stores in the body, especially to the face
- Weakening bones, the result of interference with calcium absorption

- Development of cataracts
- Acne
- High blood pressure

NSAIDs

Nonsteroidal anti-inflammatory drugs (NSAIDs) are usually prescribed for arthritis and muscle and joint pain associated with lupus, although there are over-the-counter forms available as well. Examples of NSAIDs include acetylsalicylic acid (aspirin), ibuprofen (Motrin), indomethacin (Indocin), nabumetone (Relafen), naproxen (Naprosyn), and tolmetin (Tolectin). Use of NSAIDs can cause stomach pain, stomach bleeding, dizziness, blurred vision, and kidney problems. A newer form of NSAIDs, called COX-2 inhibitors (Celebrex and Vioxx) cause slightly less stomach upset than traditional NSAIDs.

The use of NSAIDs in people with lupus can be especially dangerous. These drugs can reduce blood flow to the kidneys and cause new or further damage to these organs, as they are often already stressed and inflamed from the disease.

Antimalarials

The most widely prescribed drug in this group of drugs with anti-inflammatory properties is hydroxychloroquine (Plaquenil). Others include chloroquine (Aralen) and quinine. Antimalarials are most often prescribed for skin and joint symptoms of lupus. Although they are effective, it typically takes several months before their benefits can be appreciated. Side effects may include gastrointestinal distress, rash, muscle weakness, and decreased hearing. The most serious side effect, although rare, is a tendency for the drugs to accumulate in the retina, which can lead to blindness. It is recommended that you get an eye examination every six months when taking antimalarials.

Immunomodulating Drugs

Also known as cytotoxic drugs, these agents suppress the immune system and relieve inflammation. Two examples are azathioprine (Imuran) and cyclophosphamide (Cytoxan). Both drugs have been used with variable success in patients with severe lupus unresponsive to other treatments and in people who need very high doses of steroids. Immunomodulating drugs are usually reserved for people who have lupus that has affected the brain or kidneys. Side effects include anemia, low white blood cell count, hair loss, and an increased risk of infection. They may also increase the risk of infertility, damage to DNA, and developing cancer later in life.

Anticoagulants

These drugs are used to prevent blood from clotting too rapidly. Heparin, Coumadin, and aspirin are the three drugs usually prescribed. Anticoagulants are typically needed after an individual experiences a clotting episode (an embolism or thrombosis), after which they will probably stay on the medication for life.

Many people who have lupus and who are taking various drugs say they are frustrated because they need to undergo regular blood tests to monitor the disease and to anticipate changes in symptoms. Changes in blood test results may indicate when the disease is becoming active even before the individual experiences any symptoms of a flare-up. Early treatment of symptoms may help decrease the chance of permanent damage to the organs and reduce the amount of time the person will take drugs. Yet taking different drugs can exact a toll on the body by masking the problems rather than solving them, and causing side effects.

❖ EVALUATION AND TREATMENT OF LUPUS: MY APPROACH

At our Center, we take a drug-free approach to lupus. We look at the various signs and symptoms an individual has, and then decide which tests we will use to uncover the molecular (cellular) reasons they are occurring.

Juanita came to the Edelson Center with a long list of symptoms. She had been diagnosed with lupus nine years earlier at the age of twenty-seven. "I've taken all the drugs I can stand," she said. "Methotrexate, prednisone, Indocin, and then Imuran. I couldn't tolerate the Imuran at all. I'm so tired of being sick, and sick of being tired. I don't have the energy to take care of my four-year-old daughter, and I certainly can't go back to work."

Evaluating Juanita

Juanita's environmental history showed that she had been exposed to cigarette smoke during her entire childhood (both her parents smoked), but fortunately she did not take up the habit. After graduating from high school she had gone to work for a printing company, where she was exposed to many different chemicals, even though she worked in the front-office area. She had been promoted to account executive near her thirty-fourth birthday, but six months later she was too sick to work, so she had to quit. When Juanita came to me she was experiencing joint pain, chest pain, tight chest, fatigue, muscle pain, insomnia, rash, eczema, butterfly facial rash, twitches, itchy eyes, ear pain, ankle swelling, heartburn, constipation, shortness of breath, diarrhea, and brain fog. These symptoms suggested lupus and that several bodily systems were affected—specifically cardiac and gastrointestinal—so I chose the following tests to confirm the diagnosis and to get a complete picture of her autoimmune process:

- Antinuclear antibody (ANA) test, which was positive, thus indicating lupus.
- Anti-DNA (double-stranded DNA) test, also positive and indicating lupus.
- Echocardiogram, performed because of her chest symptoms. It showed pericardial effusion (leakage of fluid around the heart), which is often seen in people who have lupus or rheumatoid arthritis.
- Lactulose mannitol challenge, which tests for intestinal permeability. The results indicated the intestinal lining was compromised, which was likely a cause of her abdominal and intestinal problems, as well as malabsorption.
- Heavy metal challenge, which showed high levels of mercury and elevated lead and arsenic.
- Toxic chemical levels, which showed blood levels of toluene, hexane, pentane, and tetrachloroethylene, chemicals that can be found in inks and paper.
- Biochemical profile and CBC, which showed low albumin and hematocrit and high globulin, all indicating anemia. About 71 percent of people with SLE are anemic. She also had a low platelet count, which occurs in about 25 to 35 percent of people with SLE.
- 24-hour urine analysis, which showed increased loss of protein and hematuria (blood in the urine), both common in lupus patients.
- Stool test, which showed intestinal candidiasis, a frequent finding in lupus patients.

- Nutritional studies, which showed marginal deficiencies in vitamins A, C, E, B_6, and B_{12}, as well as zinc, magnesium, and several amino acids. These findings supported the problems of malabsorption indicated on her lactulose mannitol challenge.

Juanita's ANA and anti-DNA test results, along with her symptoms, confirmed the diagnosis of lupus. She also had:

- Nutritional deficiencies, malabsorption syndrome, and intestinal candidiasis, which were working together to cause her alternating diarrhea and constipation.
- Autoimmune vasculitis (inflammation of the blood vessels) with neuropathy, which means that the inflammation was affecting nerve function.
- Severe proteinuria, or the presence of protein (albumin) in the urine. This condition occurs in many patients who have lupus, and grows worse as the disease progresses. Juanita's low blood albumin level was a clue to this condition.
- Hypocorticism, a condition in which the adrenal glands do not produce enough adrenocortical hormones, which causes weakness, anemia, sluggishness, mental changes, and other symptoms. Hypocorticism is often seen in people who have lupus, as well as those with CFIDS or autoimmune thyroid conditions.
- Food and inhalant allergies. These are common among people who have lupus and, indeed, among most people who have autoimmunity. Juanita was allergic to legumes (e.g., green peas and chickpeas), and she reacted to many other different foods, including cooked cabbage, garlic, and turnips (all of which contain sulfur), as well as cigarette smoke.

Treatment

Once we identify the specific autoimmune components for a particular patient, we can begin treatment. The goal of treatment is to eliminate toxins from the body, provide the body with the nutritional components it needs to heal, deal with organ damage, and reduce the hyperactivity of the immune system. I choose the treatments based on the individual's symptoms, history, and the state of his or her immune system, which means no two patients have the same treatment program.

For Juanita, I chose the following treatment program. Hers was a very aggressive approach; not everyone needs this level of therapy. However, it gives you an idea of the possibilities. Remember, too, that there are steps you can turn to yourself (see chapters 11–13 and the end of this chapter).

• Gamma globulin. We gave Juanita megadoses of intravenous gamma globulin for several weeks, then once every two weeks for two months to help reduce inflammation. This treatment is also believed to help reduce the production of some autoantibodies and has been shown to be beneficial in kidney injuries.

• Nutritional therapy. Juanita was started on antioxidant and amino acid therapy, along with other supplements, to aid her detoxification processes. Because she was taking both DMPS and DMSA, which unavoidably remove vital minerals from the body, she was given high levels of zinc, copper, magnesium, and manganese along with her antioxidants and B vitamins during her stay at the Center and then a revised supplement program for when she returned home.

• Intravenous ozone therapy. Ozone boosts the ability of the immune system to destroy infectious organisms (specifically, candida, in Juanita's case) and improves the efficiency of antioxidant enzymes, which Juanita was receiving as part of her nutritional program to facilitate detoxification.

• Oral transfer factor. We gave Juanita this immune system modulator for six months to help balance the activity of her immune system as she went through detoxification.

• Chelation with DMSA and DMPS. Juanita was started on twice-weekly oral DMSA and once-weekly intravenous DMPS while she was at the Center, to help eliminate the heavy metals from her body. Once she left the Center she continued the oral DMSA and received the injections of DMPS from a physician near her hometown. She continued chelation for six months.

• High-temperature sauna therapy. Juanita underwent four weeks of high-temperature sauna treatments at our Center and then continued the treatments at home, once a day, for the next five months. This treatment helped remove the many chemicals we found in her bloodstream.

• Growth hormone. Although growth hormone levels decline naturally with age, Juanita's levels were below average for her age. Abnormally low levels are associated with fatigue, reduced muscle and bone strength, and other symptoms of lupus.

• Erythropoietin. This hormone is naturally secreted by the kidneys. Juanita had low erythropoietin levels, so we gave her an injectable form of the hormone to treat her anemia, because erythropoietin stimulates the production of red blood cells.

• Thymus injections. Thymus injections helped Juanita's immune system produce T-cells, which are involved in locating, identifying, and destroying antigens. This treatment has also been shown to balance the immune system.

• Avoidance diet. Once we identified Juanita's food allergies, she made some changes in her diet. She eliminated all legumes, and, to prevent the possibility that she would eat beef from alfalfa-fed cattle (beef cattle are commonly fed this legume), she also eliminated all beef and beef products. She also stopped eating foods that contain sulfur, which include onions, garlic, horseradish, brussels sprouts, and radishes.

• Environmental controls. Juanita was advised to install HEPA filters in her home and to replace household cleaning supplies with natural cleaners (e.g., vinegar, borax, lemon, baking soda). In addition to avoiding any contact with cigarette smoke, Juanita was advised to avoid fabric, carpet, and furniture stores (because of the chemicals emitted by these products) and newly painted and carpeted areas. She was also advised to follow, as much as possible, a whole foods, organic diet and to install water filters in her home.

• Pancreatic enzymes. Juanita had a deficiency of pancreatic enzymes, which are needed to help with the digestion of food. Her deficiency was a cause of her malabsorption. Juanita received daily supplements of pancreatic enzymes to help alleviate this condition.

After six months of treatment, Juanita said she "felt like a new person." Her ANA and double-stranded DNA levels had dropped dramatically, and her thyroid antibodies were in the normal range. Her muscle and joint pain was nearly gone, she had no trouble with diarrhea or constipation, and she had lots of energy. She was offered a job at her old printing office, but rather than work at the facility, she opted to work at home on her computer and telecommute so she would avoid the chemical exposure.

❖ WHAT YOU CAN DO NOW

• Find a doctor who performs the tests and uses the treatments discussed in this chapter (see chapter 2).

- Make your home environment as toxin-free as possible (see chapter 11 for specific suggestions). I recommend installation of HEPA filters and water filters, and avoidance of all pesticides, insecticides, herbicides, and household cleaning chemicals.
- Switch to a whole foods, and an organic diet that includes lots of fruits and vegetables and whole grains. You want to avoid hormones, steroids, and food additives, preservatives, and colorings (see chapter 12).
- Ask your doctor to test you for food allergies.
- At the discretion of your healthcare provider use one or more of the herbal chelators (burdock root, dandelion root, lemon balm, milk thistle, uva ursi, yellow dock) listed in chapter 11. Always consult with your healthcare provider before using herbs. I do not recommend the use of these herbs as the only biodetoxification approach.
- Consider using the nutritional chelators (glutathione, lipoic acid, cysteine, N-acetylcysteine) listed in chapter 11. Always consult with your physician before taking these supplements to determine the proper dosage and which ones are most appropriate for you.
- Take antioxidants and other essential nutrients. You can see a list of the suggested supplements and dosages in chapter 12.
- Talk to your doctor about taking DHEA (see chapter 13). This hormone should only be taken under a doctor's supervision and with periodic blood tests to monitor your DHEA levels.

Chapter 5

Autoimmune Thyroid Disorders

Of all the autoimmune diseases, those affecting the thyroid are the most common. It is estimated that as many as 10 percent of Americans have a thyroid disease. Not every thyroid condition has its roots in autoimmunity, but the majority appear to be caused by the body attacking its own thyroid glands. In this chapter we explore only those thyroid conditions that are the result of an autoimmune process and discuss what you can do if you are among those Americans whose thyroid gland is under attack.

❖ AUTOIMMUNE THYROID DISORDERS TODAY

Too much of a good thing, or too little. That sums up the basis of the two most common autoimmune thyroid disorders. On the too-much side is Graves' disease, whose main characteristic is hyperthyroidism—excess production of thyroxine, a thyroid hormone often referred to as T4. On the too-little side is Hashimoto's thyroiditis, characterized by hypothyroidism, or insufficient thyroxine. Graves' disease affects about 1 percent of

Americans (2.5 million people), while Hashimoto's thyroiditis affects between 4 and 5 percent (up to 12.5 million).

Who gets autoimmune thyroid disorders? Although people of any age can develop them, Graves' disease and Hashimoto's thyroiditis generally first appear between the ages of twenty and forty, and they affect women seven to eight times more often than men. Of these two conditions, children are more likely to get Hashimoto's thyroiditis, which can stunt their growth and so requires immediate treatment.

The Main Autoimmune Thyroid Disorders

Graves' disease is the most common type of hyperthyroidism (the overproduction of thyroid hormone). Because thyroid hormone regulates many bodily functions, overproduction can cause many serious problems, including high blood pressure, weight loss, and rapid heartbeat. Other signs associated with Graves' disease include goiter and exophthalmos (bulging eyes).

Hashimoto's thyroiditis is the most common type of hypothyroidism, a condition characterized by the underproduction of thyroid hormone. This results in a slowed metabolism, weight gain, and other symptoms. Hashimoto's thyroiditis is a type of hypothyroidism that has autoimmunity roots.

Transient thyroiditis includes postpartum thyroiditis (transient hyperthyroidism followed by transient hypothyroidism) and silent thyroiditis (transient hyperthyroidism followed by normal thyroid function). Postpartum thyroiditis usually occurs a few months after

---

childbirth and eventually resolves itself. The chance of recurrence in subsequent pregnancies is 70 percent. In transient thyroiditis, an excessive amount of thyroid hormone is released, but then eventually returns to normal. It occurs in both men and women. The good news is, therapy is usually not needed for transient thyroiditis. For that reason, we don't discuss it any further in this book.

❖ WHY SOME THYROID DISEASES ARE AUTOIMMUNE

If you have Graves' disease, your body produces autoantibodies that attack the proteins on the surface of thyroid cells. The cells respond by producing too much thyroid hormone, which overstimulates all the cells in the body and results in hyperthyroidism. What makes the hyperthyroidism associated with Graves' disease different from "regular" hyperthyroidism is the presence of the antibodies and their action against the thyroid. In "regular" hyperthyroidism, the mechanism of action is different.

In Hashimoto's thyroiditis, scientists believe autoantibodies attack several different elements of the thyroid—thyroglobulin and thyroid peroxidase—causing inflammation and reducing thyroxine production. We mention these two elements because the presence of their antibodies in the blood can be used to help diagnose Hashimoto's thyroiditis (see "Diagnosis and Treatment of Autoimmune Thyroid Disorders: Conventional Approach," on p. 106).

An interesting and unexplained feature of Graves' disease and Hashimoto's thyroiditis is that if you have Graves' disease for a while and you don't undergo treatment, your condition can transform into Hashimoto's thyroiditis. This change can work both ways.

❖ CAUSES, TRIGGERS, AND RISK FACTORS

As with most autoimmune conditions, genetics and environmental factors are believed to be the main causative factors, with each contributing. Because the factors behind Graves' disease and Hashimoto's thyroiditis seem to be similar, we look at these two conditions together, while pointing out the differences.

Genetics

Grady went to her doctor complaining of low energy, weight gain, depression, anxiety, and head palpitations. Because the symptoms suggested hypothyroidism (Hashimoto's thyroiditis), her doctor conducted thyroid tests (see "Diagnosis and Treatment of Autoimmune Thyroid Disorders: Conventional Approach," on p. 106) but found no evidence to support his suspicions. He wrote a prescription for an antidepressant and sent Grady home. A few days later she returned to her doctor, telling him that she had just learned from her mother that her grandmother and two aunts had both experienced the same symptoms around the same age (Grady was forty) and that they had improved after taking thyroid hormones. Grady was given a prescription for thyroid hormones, and within three weeks she felt much better and continued to improve.

Having a sibling, parent, grandparent, or other blood relatives with thyroid disease greatly increases your risk for getting a similar disease. It is also common for people to have symptoms of thyroid disease but to show no evidence on testing. However, a family history of the disease or other autoimmune conditions can be the deciding factor in making a diagnosis in such cases, which can then be confirmed by giving the individual a trial of thyroid medication. It is also known that if you have an identical twin who has Graves' disease, you have a 50 percent chance of developing the disease as well.

Environmental Factors

The number of cases of autoimmune thyroid problems—and other autoimmune diseases—has been rising steadily over the past few decades, and that increase is believed to be due in large part to the rising levels of toxic chemicals in our food, water, and air. These foreign substances invade our bodies and promote free radicals, placing stress on the immune system and triggering autoimmunity in susceptible individuals.

In the book *Our Stolen Future*, the authors Colburn, Dumanosky, and Myers explain how the synthetic chemicals that pollute our environment are extremely disruptive to the delicate balance of thyroid hormones. In particular, they name pesticides (herbicides, insecticides, nematocides, fungicides) that are being sent into the environment at a rate of hundreds of tons a day in the United States and around the world. Many of these pesticides contain PCBs (polychlorinated biphenyls, often found in insecticides) and dioxins (found in herbicides and Agent Orange). The authors believe these toxics disrupt the immune system and cause it to become overreactive, which in turn causes autoimmunity and thus leads to an unbalanced hormonal system. Studies suggest that PCBs are responsible for many cases of autoimmune thyroid conditions and that such problems are much more common in communities that are polluted with toxic chemicals left behind in toxic dumps or coming from active industrial plants.

Iodine is also known to trigger Graves' disease. High intake of iodide can be a factor in developed countries like the United States where people consume a lot of salt and salty foods. Thus in people susceptible to Graves' disease, excess iodide may be a problem.

Some scientists believe severe emotional stress triggers Graves' disease, yet many people get the disease without going through such an experience. Other factors that may trigger Graves' disease include mercury, lead, toxic chemicals, smoking, radiation to the neck, certain drugs (such as alpha interferon and interleukin-2), and infectious organisms.

Could microorganisms be a cause of autoimmune thyroid disease? Some researchers think so. A Greek study published in 2001 reported that the presence of antibodies to the bacteria *Yersinia enterocolitica* was fourteen times higher in people with Hashimoto's thyroiditis than in healthy individuals. Whether *Yersinia* or other microorganisms are involved in autoimmune thyroid disease has not been determined, but it is another area to be studied, as is being done in other autoimmune conditions.

❖ SIGNS AND SYMPTOMS

Graves' disease and Hashimoto's thyroiditis share common triggers, but their signs and symptoms are not the same. Here are the distinguishing factors for both of these autoimmune thyroid conditions.

Graves' Disease

This thyroid condition was named after Robert Graves, M.D., who first described this form of hyperthyroidism in 1835 in six women. Graves' disease usually comes on slowly, building over weeks or months. The first symptoms are usually weight loss and a feeling of being very anxious as the extra thyroid hormones circulating through the body speed up metabolism. Many women are glad for the weight loss, but then other symptoms appear, such as weakness, hair loss, trembling, diarrhea, and insomnia. Blood pressure and heart rate can increase to dangerous levels, and many people find they cannot tolerate heat and thus they perspire more.

Perhaps the most characteristic sign of Graves' disease is exophthalmos, or bulging of the eyes, caused by inflammation of the tissues behind the eyeball. This condition occurs in about 50 percent of people who have Graves' disease. The inflammation is believed to be caused by autoantibodies that attack the eye tissues. Exophthalmos is often accompanied by blurred or reduced vision, double vision, and red eyes. Fortunately this inflammation looks worse than it is, because 99 percent of the time it does not cause permanent or serious damage.

Another characteristic sign of Graves' disease is an enlarged thyroid, or goiter. Often individuals notice they are having trouble swallowing, which is a clue to the enlargement, or they may feel a lump when they touch the front of their neck.

Other symptoms of Graves' disease include:

- Fatigue
- Sweaty palms
- Fine, brittle hair
- Restlessness
- Depression
- Increased appetite
- Change in sex drive
- Irregular menstrual cycle (in women)
- Reduced attention span

Hashimoto's Thyroiditis

Do you feel cold even when everyone else is warm and comfortable? Is your skin very dry and flaking, and are your nails thin and brittle? Are you pale? Then you may have Hashimoto's thyroiditis, the most common cause of hypothyroidism. Teresa was experiencing all these symptoms, and at first she chalked it up to overwork. She was working full-time as a marketing representative and, at age forty-one, had just started taking classes at night to get her master's degree. "Then I began to gain weight, and I couldn't understand why," said Teresa. "I certainly wasn't eating more; in fact I didn't even have time to eat sometimes. I didn't understand what was happening."

Teresa went to her doctor, who said she was probably just under stress and going through premenopause. He sent her home with a prescription for an antidepressant, which she refused to take because she didn't believe depression was her problem. After several months, her symptoms got worse, and she could barely drag herself to class at night. Fortunately, Teresa decided to go to an endocrinologist (a doctor who specializes in gland disorders), who recognized the symptoms of a slowed metabolism, and after a series of tests (see "Diagnosis and Treatment of Autoimmune Thyroid Disorders: Conventional Approach," below) she was diagnosed with Hashimoto's thyroiditis.

Other symptoms of Hashimoto's thyroiditis include swelling of bodily tissues, the result of fluid accumulation that accompanies weight gain. Swelling can occur both internally and externally, especially around the eyes. A slow metabolism also means digestive processes are reduced, which often leads to severe constipation. Other symptoms of Hashimoto's thyroiditis include:

- Fatigue, the result of slowed muscle function and muscle pain that make it harder, and thus more tiresome, to perform normal activities).
- Slowed heartbeat and reduced blood flow to muscles, which contribute to feelings of tiredness.
- Decreased ability to concentrate and to solve problems.
- Decreased interest in relationships and activities.

When Hashimoto's occurs in children, it is especially important to get treatment immediately, because it can slow growth.

❖ DIAGNOSIS AND TREATMENT OF AUTOIMMUNE THYROID DISORDERS: CONVENTIONAL APPROACH

Like most other autoimmune conditions, autoimmune thyroid disorders can be difficult to diagnose. Some people have obvious signs and symptoms, backed up by positive test results, but others may have only a few symptoms and negative test results, which can not only be frustrating for those individuals, but also delay proper treatment. Conventional treatment relies heavily on drugs, which people usually need to take for the rest of their lives. Taking thyroid medication can be tricky, because any significant increase or decrease in a person's metabolic rate can have a great impact on how the body processes the drugs. In Graves' disease, the body eliminates certain drugs much more quickly than usual; in Hashimoto's thyroiditis, drugs stay in the body longer. In this section, we look at how conventional doctors diagnose and treat autoimmune thyroid disorders.

Diagnosing Autoimmune Thyroid Disorders

Results of a physical examination, a thorough medical and family history, and blood tests typically are used to make diagnoses of both Graves' disease and Hashimoto's thyroiditis. If your doctor orders other, more expensive tests, such as a radioactive iodine uptake or thyroid ultrasound test, before doing blood tests, you should ask why, because blood tests can be sufficient for a diagnosis. Here are the blood tests and what they can tell you.

- Thyroxine (T4) levels. This blood test reveals the amount of this hormone secreted by the thyroid gland. Elevated levels suggest hyperthyroidism; abnormally low levels suggest hypothyroidism.
- Free T4 test. This test is more sophisticated, and more expensive, than the T4 test. It can be used to diagnose both hyper- and hypothyroidism.
- Thyroid-stimulating hormone (TSH) levels. Low blood levels of TSH are the most reliable test for hyperthyroidism; high levels indicate hypothyroidism.
- Antithyroid peroxidase (anti-TPO) antibody test. Elevated levels of this antibody are often seen in people who have Hashimoto's thyroiditis.

Several nonblood tests also may be needed. One that is sometimes done when Graves' disease is suspected is measurement of radioactive iodine uptake. High uptake indicates Graves' disease, while low uptake points to various other thyroid conditions, including subacute or granulomatous thyroiditis (a painful condition believed to be caused by a virus), iodine-induced hyperthyroidism, silent thyroiditis, and postpartum thyroiditis.

Sometimes an individual has an enlarged thyroid, negative

results on antibody testing, and suspicious nodules. In such cases, doctors may do a fine-needle aspiration biopsy, in which a needle is inserted into the thyroid to get a tissue sample to identify Hashimoto's thyroiditis, thyroid cysts, benign adenomas, and other conditions.

Oops: Misdiagnosing Autoimmune Thyroid Disease

- Although bulging eyes are a classic sign of Graves' disease, not everyone who has bulging eyes has this thyroid condition (and not everyone who has Graves' disease has bulging eyes). Bulging eyes may also be caused by severe nearsightedness, certain liver dysfunctions, drugs such as cortisone, and losing or gaining a lot of weight.

- Elevated thyroxine levels are a common sign of Graves' disease, but other factors that can raise these levels include oral contraceptives, pregnancy, hepatitis, and postmenopausal estrogen treatments.

- Some symptoms of Hashimoto's thyroiditis can be confused with those of depression. When some doctors see these symptoms (lack of interest in activities, decreased ability to concentrate) in women, they tend to diagnose depression without looking further.

- Although rare (occurring in less than 5 percent of people who have hypothyroidism), other causes of low levels of TSH need to be ruled out in order to diagnose Hashimoto's thyroiditis. They include pituitary gland or hypothalamic problems, or problems with the adrenal glands or ovaries.

Treating Graves' Disease

Before a formal treatment program is chosen, most doctors initially recommend a "quick fix"—a beta-adrenergic blocking drug (beta-blocker), such as atenolol (Tenormin), metoprolol (Lopressor), nadolol (Corgard), or propranolol (Inderal). These drugs block the effects of circulating thyroid hormone in the body, reduce nervousness, and slow the heart rate in as little as a few hours. (If you have asthma, insulin-dependent diabetes, or a heart condition, however, these drugs should not be used.) Then the doctor may choose from the following choices:

• Antithyroid drugs such as propylthiouracil (PTU) and methimazole (Tapazole) are usually prescribed for children, young people, elderly people who have a heart condition, or for people who have mild Graves' disease. These drugs make it difficult for the body to use the iodine required to make thyroid hormone, which in turn reduces production of the hormone. These drugs result in long-term remission in only about 20 to 30 percent of people. About 5 percent of people who take these drugs develop a rash, hives, fever, or joint pain. In rare cases, white blood cell levels drop, which reduces a person's ability to resist infection. This condition can be fatal in some people.

Because available drugs cannot cure this disease, the goal of medication is remission. Most doctors tell their patients that if they have not achieved remission after two to four years of treatment, they probably never will. That's when another treatment choice is usually presented to patients: radioactive iodine.

• Radioactive iodine (RAI) can be taken as a capsule or a liquid. The iodine travels from the stomach to the bloodstream and into the thyroid gland. Because the thyroid gland needs iodine to make thyroid hormone, it readily accepts the RAI. However, the radiation destroys some of the thyroid cells, which in turn reduces production of the thyroid hormone. The RAI eventually becomes nonradioactive and leaves the body in urine. A big problem with RAI, however, is that because the amount of damage it does cannot be controlled, at least 50 percent of people who take RAI eventually develop hypothyroidism, usually within ten years. These individuals then must be treated with a thyroid hormone supplement (see below). Essentially, they've traded one disorder for another, yet many doctors justify using this approach because hyperthyroidism is more dangerous than hypothyroidism, so patients are left with the lesser of two evils—and medication they must take for the rest of their lives.

A more drastic approach is thyroid ablative surgery, in which part of the thyroid is destroyed using radioactive iodine. The result is less thyroid tissue, which means less activity and less hormone production. Surgery is usually reserved for people who have very large goiters or for children or adolescents who have not responded to antithyroid drug therapy.

Treating Hashimoto's Thyroiditis

Doctors do not always agree on the best course of treatment for the early stages of this disease. Some doctors recommend a watch-and-wait approach, using blood tests periodically to monitor TPO antibodies and T3 levels to see if the condition worsens. Others start thyroid hormone treatment immediately. Because the chance of remission is less than 10 percent, more doctors choose the drug approach. The most frequently used thyroid treatment is synthetic thyroxine (e.g., Synthroid, Levothroid, Levo-T), which triggers the normal body's response of generating

T3. It also leads to normal levels of TSH and normal thyroid gland functioning, often within a few weeks.

As with any thyroid medication, dosages need to be monitored carefully and changed as needed. Stress, illness, physical trauma, surgical procedures, and menopause can all have an effect on the amount of medication the body needs to regulate the thyroid, so it is common for doctors to periodically adjust dosage levels.

❖ EVALUATION AND TREATMENT OF AUTOIMMUNE THYROID DISORDERS: MY APPROACH

Along with a physical examination and the thyroid tests used by conventional physicians, my approach to evaluation of people with autoimmune thyroid disorders includes a thorough environmental history. The thyroid gland is very sensitive to the impact of environmental pollutants, which can disrupt metabolism. For this reason, a person's environmental history proves to be very revealing when I do an evaluation and helps me decide which treatments to start. Rose is an example.

Evaluating Autoimmune Thyroid Disease

"Can you help me, I'm a wreck," said Rose as soon as she was seated in my office. Rose looked older than her fifty-two years: her hair was brittle, thinning, and lacked luster, and her skin was very dry, accenting her wrinkles. Her fingers trembled slightly, and her entire body seemed charged with energy. Yet, said Rose, she was always tired. "My insides are revved up, but my body is weak," she explained. She complained of insomnia, diarrhea, sweaty hands, and depression.

Rose's environmental history revealed various toxic exposures. Although she did not smoke herself, she had been married for seventeen years to a man who smoked two packs a day (she was now divorced). She had worked part-time for nearly twenty years at a plant nursery, where she was exposed to pesticides and fertilizers. She also had six amalgams that she had had done during her teenage years and that were still intact.

Rose's thyroid was enlarged, and with her other symptoms I suspected Graves' disease, even though she did not have bulging eyes, seen in about 50 percent of people with Graves'. I ran the comprehensive thyroid autoantibody study, and test results showed elevated levels of thyroxine (T4) and free T4, abnormally low levels of TSH, low antithyroglobulin antibodies (ATAs), and a positive result on the radioactive iodine uptake test. She also had elevated thyroid peroxidase enzymes and positive antinuclear antibodies (ANAs). Heavy metal challenge showed mercury, and a chemical toxicity test showed benzene, formaldehyde, and several pesticides. "My last doctor said I was just going through menopause and that I shouldn't worry so much," she said. "He didn't even check my thyroid."

Treating Rose

We started Rose on the antithyroid medication methimazole and a detoxification and treatment program that included:

• Chelation with DMSA and DMPS to remove mercury. She started chelation at the Center and then returned many times to complete her treatments.

• High-temperature sauna to remove the chemicals in her bloodstream. She started her program at the Center and then continued it at home daily for five months in a home sauna.

• Transfer factor was started at a high dose and gradually reduced over a four-month period. The benefit of transfer factor is that it modulates function of the immune system, bringing it into balance.

• Thymus extracts. Within two weeks of starting thymus extracts, Rose saw a significant improvement in her skin and hair, which we attributed largely to the thymus extracts.

• Antioxidant therapy was prescribed to help eliminate free radicals and to help the thyroid function better. Rose was prescribed high doses of beta-carotene, vitamin C, vitamin E, coenzyme Q10, lipoic acid, and the bioflavonoids quercetin and pygnogenol.

• Environmental controls were recommended, including installation of HEPA filters in her home (she did put one in her bedroom), reverse-osmosis carbon filters for her water, a switch to organic foods whenever possible, avoidance of cigarette smoke, and avoidance of circumstances in which chemicals are typically present, including buildings with new furniture, paint, carpeting, and other renovations; stores that sell furniture, carpeting, wood products, fabrics, and building supplies; and nursery and agricultural settings in which pesticides and other chemicals are used. Fortunately, she no longer worked at the nursery.

• Nutritional therapy. Because people with Graves' disease have a rapid metabolism, they don't absorb as many nutrients from their food. Thus, not only is the food they eat important, but they need nutritional supplementation as well. Omega-3 and omega-6 fatty acids are especially important, as they help suppress thyroid functioning. To get these essential fatty acids, Rose took both fish oil and flaxseed oil daily. Minerals are critical for thyroid functioning, so Rose was prescribed a multivitamin-mineral that contained 25 mg zinc, 1 mg copper, and 200 mcg selenium. In addition, she took 200 mcg chromium, 1200 mg calcium, and 400 mg magnesium.

• Dietary suggestions. Foods that help suppress thyroid functioning include pears, peaches, cruciferous vegetables (brussels sprouts, cauliflower, broccoli, cabbage, and others), and spinach. Overall, a diet that is low in fat, animal protein, refined sugar, and salt is recommended, and I urged Rose to follow that plan.

After six months of treatment, Rose said she felt, and looked, younger. Her skin, hair, and nails had improved dramatically. She had much of her energy back, but without the "revved up" feeling she had experienced in the past. Depression and insomnia were no longer a problem.

Treating Hashimoto's Thyroiditis

My treatment approach to Hashimoto's thyroiditis is similar to that for Graves' disease—chelation and high-temperature sauna for detoxification, transfer factor, thymus extracts, and antioxidants. I also add low-dose thyroid medication rather than an antithyroid drug, and perhaps an anti-inflammatory, such as ibuprofen, to reduce thyroid inflammation.

❖ WHAT YOU CAN DO NOW

Here are some ways to deal with both types of autoimmune thyroid conditions:

• Avoid tap water, which contains fluoride and chlorine. These substances block the thyroid's iodine receptors, which causes a decreased production of hormone containing iodine. This condition is associated with hypothyroidism, so you can exacerbate your situation if you consume these substances.
• Because hypothyroidism is the opposite of hyperthyroidism, the foods that help Graves' disease should be eaten in

moderation or avoided if you have Hashimoto's thyroiditis (See "Treating Rose"). However, foods that may be helpful include dates, apricots, prunes, and fish.

• Avoid table salt. According to Edward Bauman, Ph.D., Associate Dean of Nutrition at the University of Natural Medicine in New Mexico, commercial iodized salt contains aluminum and sugar, which irritate the thyroid and can cause imbalances. Instead, people are urged to use Celtic Sea Salt, Japanese salt, or sea salt, which can be found in health food stores.

• Establish a strong support network of family, friends, or others with similar conditions. People with autoimmune thyroid conditions are typically extremely sensitive people, and so having emotional as well as physical support is critical for their well-being (see appendix).

• Find a doctor who performs the tests and uses the treatments discussed in this chapter (see chapter 2).

• Make your home environment as toxin-free as possible (see chapter 11 for specific suggestions). I recommend installation of HEPA filters and water filters, and avoidance of all pesticides, insecticides, herbicides, and household cleaning chemicals.

• Switch to a whole foods, organic diet that includes lots of fruits and vegetables and whole grains. You want to avoid hormones, steroids, and food additives, preservatives, and colorings (see chapter 12).

• Use one or more of the herbal chelators (burdock root, dandelion root, lemon balm, milk thistle, uva ursi, yellow dock; at the discretion of your healthcare provider) listed in chapter 11. Always consult with your healthcare provider before using herbs. I do not recommend use of these herbs as the only biodetoxification approach.

• Consider using the nutritional chelators (glutathione, lipoic acid, cysteine, N-acetylcysteine) listed in chapter 11. Always consult with your physician before taking these supplements to determine the proper dosage and which ones are most appropriate for you.

• Take antioxidants and other essential nutrients. You can see a list of the suggested supplements and dosages in chapter 12.

Chapter 6

Rheumatoid Arthritis

Rheumatoid arthritis is an autoimmune disease in which the immune system attacks primarily the joints but also various other parts of the body. Although this disease was only "officially" recognized by the medical community during the 1800s, it did not suddenly appear on the scene just a few short centuries ago. Archaeologists have found evidence of rheumatoid arthritis in bones that are thousands of years old, indicating that this autoimmune disease has ancient roots.

For example, the bones of Roman emperor Constantine IX (A.D. 980–1055) have evidence of rheumatoid arthritis, as do several Native American skeletons dating from 6500 to 450 B.C. found along the Tennessee River. A few skeletons found in Mexico dating from 140 B.C. to A.D. 1550 also show signs of the deformities caused by rheumatoid arthritis, although no signs have been detected in ancient bones found in Europe and Asia. So why was rheumatoid arthritis considered to be a "new" disease in the 1800s, when it has been around since ancient times?

The reasons are simple: age and environmental factors. The

vast majority of our ancestors did not live long enough to get the disease—but we do. Until just a few short centuries ago, most people did not live past the age of thirty, which is the approximate age at which the disease strikes. And our ancestors were not exposed to the toxins that are pumped into our air, water, and soil, a practice that began with the industrial revolution around 1780. That practice has escalated to the point where millions of tons of pollutants are sent into our environment every day. These toxins cause the formation of free radicals, ready to invade our bodies and trigger the autoimmune process. As for the evidence of rheumatoid arthritis found in ancient people, scientists believe those isolated cases can be attributed to an infectious agent confined to isolated populations.

❖ RHEUMATOID ARTHRITIS TODAY

Several years ago, Margaret would nearly bound out of bed in the morning. She was a whirlwind of activity, taking a brisk walk every morning before breakfast, then hurrying off to work at a florist for eight hours, then home to her own flowers and ever-expanding herb gardens. At forty-one she was tired of working for other people and was in the midst of writing a business plan to open her own organic herb nursery and shop. One or two nights a week she went country dancing with friends. She experienced some aches and pains, but she didn't worry about them.

But within the next few years, those aches and pains blossomed into swelling, inflammation, limited mobility, and stiffness in the joints in her hands and knees. Now, at forty-five, it takes her several minutes to ease herself out of bed in the morning. Gone are the brisk walks and weekly country dancing outings with her friends. "The worst part is the pain and stiffness in my hands and fingers," says Margaret. "This condition has shattered my dream of having my own herb business, because I wanted to get my hands dirty and do a lot of the planting and growing myself. That's the part I love. But my hands won't let me do that now."

Margaret is among the approximately 2.5 million Americans who suffer with rheumatoid arthritis. Worldwide it affects 1 to 2 percent of the general population. More than 60 percent of those affected are women. Although the disease can strike at any age, it usually starts in young adulthood, between years twenty and forty-five.

Because the disease first strikes people when they are young and starting families and developing careers, it can have a dramatic effect on self-esteem, career advancement, financial opportunities, and relationships. And the impact can be devastating: one survey reveals that 70 percent of people with rheumatoid arthritis say the disease prevents them from living a fully productive life. Margaret certainly agrees with that statement.

So does Joseph, a forty-one-year-old former construction worker, whose arthritis prevented him from continuing in his trade. "I'd done construction work since I was a teenager," he said. "But the arthritis made it impossible for me to continue, so I had to take a sales job, making a lot less money." People like Margaret and Joseph have had their lives turned around because their immune systems have gone awry, caught up in the auto-immune process.

❖ RHEUMATOID ARTHRITIS: THE AUTOIMMUNE PROCESS

Under normal circumstances, as the immune system fights invaders, disease-fighting white blood cells—T-cells, B-cells, and leukocytes—gather at an injured or infected site, causing inflammation. The inflammatory process is usually controlled and self-limiting, dissipating as the immune cells complete their task and promote healing. But in people who have rheumatoid arthritis, the inflammatory process keeps going. For reasons that are not entirely clear, the T-cells mistake the body's own collagen cells as invaders and try to get rid of the perceived threat. The B-cells are then stimulated to produce autoantibodies, which attack the body's own tissue. The autoantibodies in rheumatoid arthritis are known as rheumatoid factors, and they primarily attack the joints, causing inflammation, stiffness, and pain.

The leukocytes are then spurred into action by the T-cells. They promote inflammation and also produce large amounts of cytokines, which are believed to have a critical role in joint damage and inflammation, and to cause fever and organ damage. One important type of cytokine you may want to remember is the tumor necrosis factor, which is the subject of much research (see "Diagnosis and Treatment of Rheumatoid Arthritis: Conventional Approach"). Levels of tumor necrosis factor rise dramatically in the synovial fluid in the joints of people who are experiencing a flare-up of the disease.

❖ CAUSES, RISK FACTORS, AND TRIGGERS

Most scientists and doctors, myself included, agree that the autoimmune process that leads to rheumatoid arthritis is the result of a combination of factors, including genetics and environmental agents. Let's look at some of those factors and their possible role in rheumatoid arthritis.

Genetics

Scientists have identified several genetic factors that may be key players in rheumatoid arthritis. A molecule called HLA-DR4, for example, is found in about 70 percent of people who have rheumatoid arthritis. (HLA-DR4 is also found in other auto-immune disorders, which strengthens the idea of the common origins of autoimmune disorders.) Another genetic factor seen in rheumatoid arthritis is a gene known as p53, which, when mutated, may promote the formation of pannus, a growth of thickened synovial tissue that occurs in rheumatoid arthritis. However, not everyone who has rheumatoid arthritis has any one or more of these particular genes, and some people who do have these genes never develop the disease. Therefore, although scientists believe that more than one gene is involved in rheumatoid arthritis, genetics is apparently only part of the disease process.

When it comes to genetic relationships, the risk of getting rheumatoid arthritis depends on how close the affected family member is. While 1 percent of the general population can expect to get rheumatoid arthritis, people with a brother or sister who has the disease have a 2 to 4 percent chance of getting the disease, while those with an identical twin with the disease have a 12 to 15 percent chance.

Environmental Factors

• The number one environmental factor, in my opinion, is heavy metal chemical toxicity, which leads to the production of free radicals in the body. I find that most of my patients who have rheumatoid arthritis also have toxic levels of heavy metals or chemicals in their bodies. The resulting free radicals attack the joints in people predisposed to autoimmunity.

• One major theory is that a mycoplasma—a type of micro-organism that is smaller than bacteria—triggers the autoimmune process in people who are genetically susceptible to rheumatoid arthritis. *Proteus mirabilis* and *Klebsiella pneumoniae*, two types of intestinal organisms, also may be triggers. It is believed these bacteria enter the bloodstream through the intestinal lining through openings caused by leaky gut syndrome. Leaky gut syndrome, or intestinal permeability, is a condition in which the intestinal lining has unusually large pores that allow toxic substances such as bacteria to enter the bloodstream. Once the bacteria are in the bloodstream, the immune system attacks them. Because these bacteria resemble antigens found in the joints, the immune system attacks the joints as well. This autoimmune process is called molecular mimicry (when part of a molecule of one protein resembles part of another totally different protein), and only occurs in individuals who have a genetic predisposition for rheumatoid arthritis.

• Diet also appears to be a factor. "Rheumatoid arthritis is not found in cultures where people eat a traditional, healthful diet high in fruits, vegetables, and fiber and low in meat, sugar, and saturated fat," says Joseph Pizzorno Jr., N.D. The disease is common, however, in American and other cultures where people eat a diet high in meat, sugar, and saturated fat and low in healthy foods. A poor diet promotes the formation of free radicals, which is the basis of autoimmunity. People with rheumatoid arthritis also often have food allergies, food sensitivities, or both. Food allergy can lead to molecular mimicry, with attacks on joints when certain foods are eaten. Exposure to foods that cause allergies and sensitivities can severely burden the immune system, promoting free-radical damage to the joints, as well as malabsorption, which occurs secondary to inflammation of the small intestine.

• Heavy smokers beware: a 2001 study published in the *Annals of the Rheumatic Diseases* reports that people who smoke a pack of cigarettes a day for more than forty years are thirteen times more likely than nonsmokers to develop rheumatoid arthritis. People who smoke less or who have smoked for fewer years also are at high risk, but less so. Although the researchers do not know the exact reason why heavy smoking is linked with rheumatoid arthritis, they do know that smoking promotes free-radical production, probably from the toxins in smoke. It appears that smoking affects the body's production of rheumatoid factor, the antibody found in many people who have rheumatoid arthritis. Other studies have also shown that exposure to smoke over time increases the body's production of these antibodies in both healthy people and those with rheumatoid arthritis.

• Hormones have been named as a possible trigger of rheumatoid arthritis, largely because women are three times more likely to get the disease than men. So far, however, scientists have not identified the hormonal factors that may be involved.

❖ SIGNS AND SYMPTOMS

At first, Cynthia thought she had the flu. Her knees and wrists were stiff first thing in the morning, and she was feverish for several weeks. She blamed her fatigue on overwork, as she was putting in about fifty hours a week as a management consultant. When her knuckles began to swell and ache, she grew worried, as her symptoms were affecting her ability to work. "My mother had had the same symptoms when she was about forty-five years old," said Cynthia. "And she was diagnosed with rheumatoid arthritis. But I didn't want to believe that it was happening to me, and I kept telling myself I was too young. But at the same time, I was so afraid that it was true and that I was going to be crippled. I was almost too afraid to go to a doctor." After several months of treating the pain and swelling with over-the-counter medications, Cynthia finally did go to a doctor, who gave her the diagnosis she had feared.

Typical Symptoms

Cynthia had many of the hallmark symptoms of rheumatoid arthritis. The official criteria for diagnosis have been defined by the Arthritis Foundation. A diagnosis requires that seven of the following eight criteria be met, with the symptoms of the first five lasting more than six weeks.

- Morning stiffness that lasts for at least one hour
- Swelling in at least one joint
- Swelling of at least one other joint
- Pain on motion in at least one joint
- Symmetrical joint swelling, not including the joint closest to the fingertips
- X-ray evidence of rheumatoid arthritis
- Lumps, or nodules, about the size of a pea, under the skin on the forearm below the elbow. These occur in about 20 to 25 percent of people with rheumatoid arthritis, usually those who have the progressive form of the disease. They are caused by inflammation of small blood vessels and are usually painless.
- Positive results on a rheumatoid factor test

The joints most often affected are the knuckles and wrist, plus the knees and the joints of the ball of the foot. Rheumatoid arthritis affects other joints less often. Swollen, painful joints often feel warm and puffy when touched. Fluid may accumulate in some joints, especially in the ankles. Rarely, fluid collects behind the knee and forms what is called Baker's cyst. This cyst feels like a tumor and is often painful.

More Than Joints

Because rheumatoid arthritis is a systemic disease, it can attack other parts of the body in addition to the joints. Fever, fatigue, and weight loss are often present during the early stages of the disease. Lesions may form on the eye, or people may develop dry eyes. The skin can become fragile and bruise easily, especially in the elderly. In some people, expanding growths in the joints can press against nerves and cause partial or total loss of function, such as a "dropped" foot or hand. Inflammation of the pericardium (the sac around the heart), spleen (splenomegaly), or lymph nodes (lymphadenopathy); obstructive lung disease; and anemia also may result from rheumatoid arthritis. Rheumatoid arthritis is associated with a higher risk for certain cancers of the blood, particularly lymphoma, which has also been associated with chemical toxicity. People with rheumatoid arthritis are also prone to infections and gastrointestinal disorders, a common feature of many autoimmune conditions.

❖ COURSE OF THE DISEASE

The course of destruction associated with rheumatoid arthritis differs for each person. For some people, the disease becomes less aggressive, and symptoms may even improve. Any deformities or damage to bones and ligaments are permanent, however. Generally, the disease course goes like this:

• A normal joint is surrounded by a joint capsule that protects it. Cartilage covers the ends of the two bones and acts as a cushion or shock absorber.

• The joint capsule is lined with a tissue called synovium, which produces synovial fluid. The fluid lubricates the cartilage and bones inside the capsule.

• In the autoimmune process of rheumatoid arthritis, the autoantibodies attack inside the joint capsule. The cells of the synovium grow abnormally, making the synovium thick, causing inflammation that results in redness, swelling, warmth, and pain.

• As the disease progresses, the abnormal synovial cells destroy the cartilage and bone inside the joint capsule.

• As the joint deteriorates, the muscles, tendons, and ligaments that surround the joint become weaker, contributing to the pain and limited mobility.

Some people experience constant symptoms; others describe a roller-coaster of events—times when they feel good (remission) and times when they feel worse. Although very few people achieve complete remission of the disease, about 50 to 70 percent remain capable of full-time employment. After fifteen to twenty years of having the disease, only 10 percent of people become invalids. Generally the average life expectancy may be shortened by three to seven years, mostly due to infection, drug side effects, and gastrointestinal bleeding.

❖ DIAGNOSIS AND TREATMENT OF RHEUMATOID ARTHRITIS: CONVENTIONAL APPROACH

Rheumatoid arthritis can be difficult to diagnose, because many other conditions mimic the symptoms of joint aches and pain (see box). Also, symptoms can develop insidiously, and conventional blood tests and X-rays may not show any abnormalities for months after joint pain has begun. This lack of clinical evidence of the disease often means that a diagnosis is delayed, which allows for further damage to occur.

That said, conventional physicians resort to several different tests to diagnose the disease. Here are the tests typically used by doctors; those your physician uses may differ.

Other Diseases That Mimic Rheumatoid Arthritis

Many other diseases and conditions mimic the symptoms of joint pain and aches associated with rheumatoid arthritis. In fact, something as simple as sleeping on a poor mattress can cause painful joints. Some people confuse rheumatoid arthritis with osteoarthritis, a condition that usually occurs in older people, is located in only one or a few joints, and causes less inflammation.

Some other conditions that may be confused with rheumatoid arthritis include the following:

Bacterial endocarditis
Behçet's disease
Chronic fatigue and immune
    deficiency syndrome
    (CFIDS)
Fibromyalgia
Gout and pseudogout
Hepatitis C
Infectious arthritis
Inflammatory bowel disease

Kawasaki's disease
Leukemia
Lupus (systemic lupus
    erythematosus)
Lyme disease
Rheumatic fever
Septic arthritis
Systemic vasculitis
Viral arthritis

Tests to Diagnose Rheumatoid Arthritis

- **Rheumatoid factor.** In about 80 percent of people diagnosed with rheumatoid arthritis, blood tests reveal rheumatoid factor (RF), antibodies that collect in the synovium of the joint.
- **Erythrocyte sedimentation rate.** An elevated rate may indicate the presence of inflammation, infection, and collagen vascular disorders.
- **C-reactive protein.** High levels of C-reactive protein in the blood indicate active inflammation.
- **X-rays.** X-rays usually are not useful in detecting early rheumatoid arthritis because they are incapable of showing images of soft tissue. A technique called dual energy X-ray absorptiometry, however, is proving to be more helpful in revealing bone loss in early-stage disease.
- **Hemoglobin and hematocrit tests.** These blood tests reveal the amount of red blood cells in the bloodstream. This is helpful for detecting anemia, which is a fairly common complication of rheumatoid arthritis.

Other Tests

Doctors may also perform the following tests if they suspect you have rheumatoid arthritis.

- Synovial fluid analysis: abnormal results may indicate the presence of rheumatoid arthritis, as well as other types of arthritis.
- Complement levels, which indicate the presence of inflammation.
- Synovial biopsy: abnormal results may indicate the presence of rheumatoid arthritis, as well as other conditions, such as fungal infection, abnormal iron levels, tumors, or cancer.

- ANA test: the presence of antinuclear antibodies in the blood can indicate rheumatoid arthritis, lupus, chronic liver disease, or scleroderma.

Treatment

Medical treatment of rheumatoid arthritis consists primarily of two types of drugs: nonsteroidal anti-inflammatory drugs (NSAIDs), which are used to suppress inflammation as much as possible to reduce the damage caused to the joints; and disease-modifying antirheumatic drugs (DMARDs), which attempt to stop or slow down the overall progression of the disease.

Although both NSAIDs and DMARDs have many side effects, those associated with DMARDs are generally considered to be more severe. For this reason, doctors have been reluctant to prescribe them until later in the course of the disease. Physicians tend to follow a pyramid approach: first they prescribe the least toxic NSAIDs and gradually build up to stronger ones, then add DMARDs as needed for relief. This entire process can take five years or longer. However, research shows that serious joint damage occurs very early in rheumatoid arthritis, which suggests that DMARDs should be started early to prevent joint damage. Many doctors, however, still prescribe NSAIDs for early disease.

PROBLEMS WITH THE PYRAMID

Some doctors argue that the side effects of NSAIDs can be just as severe as those caused by some DMARDs. Therefore, they argue that it is better to start the DMARDs early in the disease so they can help prevent joint damage, and this advantage offsets the disadvantage of the side effects caused by these drugs. Such an aggressive approach is controversial. Individuals who wish to consider it need to discuss the many undesirable effects with their physician and weigh them against the possible benefits. In my opinion, however, use of NSAIDs and DMARDs should be avoided, because they do not address the cause of rheumatoid arthritis and they are associated with many adverse effects.

NONSTEROIDAL ANTI-INFLAMMATORY DRUGS (NSAIDs)

Rheumatoid arthritis hurts, and NSAIDs are the most popular drugs to treat that pain. Among the dozens of NSAIDs available, aspirin, ibuprofen, naproxen, and ketoprofen are the most commonly used. NSAIDs block prostaglandins, substances that dilate blood vessels and cause pain and inflammation. The optimal time to take NSAIDs is upon awakening in the morning, when pain and stiffness typically peak, and after the evening meal.

If taken for long periods, NSAIDs can damage the mucous layer in the gastrointestinal system and cause bleeding. This risk exists as long as people take the drugs and up to one year after they stop. Taking NSAIDs with food can help reduce the severity of the damage, but it also reduces the potency of the drugs. Even one week of drug use can initiate bleeding in some people, especially the elderly. Buffered aspirin does not prevent bleeding. NSAIDs can also interfere with the effectiveness of other drugs taken for the disease.

Some people who take NSAIDs also take a drug to help prevent the gastrointestinal side effects. Omeprazole (Prilosec) and misoprostol (Arthrotec, Cytotec) are often used for this purpose, but they have side effects of their own, including diarrhea, cramps, and gas.

In addition to gastrointestinal effects, NSAIDs can also cause dizziness, headache, ringing in the ears, depression, rash, and kidney damage. They can increase blood pressure, especially in those who are taking medications for hypertension. Anyone who has heart problems, kidney disease, or liver problems should be monitored closely when taking NSAIDs.

A newer type of NSAID is the COX-2 (cyclooxygenase-2) inhibitor. The two drugs in this category (celecoxib [Celebrex], valdecoxib [Bextra], and rofecoxib [Vioxx]) reportedly are less likely to cause gastrointestinal problems; however, they still occur in some patients. Other problems with the COX-2 inhibitors include possible adverse effects on kidney function, especially in elderly people; a greater risk of bleeding when taking anticoagulant drugs at the same time; and a risk of higher blood levels of drugs such as methotrexate, ACE inhibitors, and warfarin.

DISEASE-MODIFYING ANTIRHEUMATIC DRUGS

While NSAIDs all work using the same mechanism—blocking the activity of prostaglandins—DMARDs have little in common except for the fact that they can slow down the progression of rheumatoid arthritis. Each of these drugs differs in exactly how it does that. The most commonly prescribed DMARDs include gold compounds, methotrexate (most prescribed of all the DMARDs), sulfasalazine, hydroxychloroquine (an antimalarial drug), and leflunomide (Arava, the newest DMARD).

Although all of these drugs can significantly delay the long-term damage associated with rheumatoid arthritis, they also all lose their effectiveness over time, usually by two years. Gastrointestinal and other side effects are common and can be very serious: nausea, vomiting, diarrhea (especially with gold), mouth sores, rash, kidney and liver damage, headache, eye damage (hydroxychloroquine), osteoporosis (methotrexate), hair loss (leflunomide), lung disease, and an increased risk for infections.

If use of a single DMARD is not effective, combinations are often prescribed. One of the drugs in combination therapy is usually methotrexate (Rheumatrex), as it works faster (within a few weeks) than other DMARDs.

Two new additions to the DMARD category of drugs have been genetically engineered to target tumor necrosis factor and other cytokines (see "Rheumatoid Arthritis: The Autoimmune Process," on p. 119). The two drugs are etanercept (Enbrel), which neutralizes tumor necrosis factor; and infliximab (Remicade), which was originally approved for Crohn's disease, another autoimmune disorder. It also works for psoriasis, another autoimmune condition.

Etanercept inhibits the progression of joint destruction in people with moderate to severe disease by neutralizing tumor necrosis factor. It can be used in combination with methotrexate in patients who do not respond adequately to methotrexate alone. Adverse effects associated with etanercept include reaction at the injection site (37 percent of patients), infections (35 percent), and headache (17 percent). Rare cases of demyelinating conditions such as multiple sclerosis and blood disorders such as aplastic anemia have occurred, as well as onset of seizure disorders. Etanercept should not be used if you have an infection.

Infliximab was approved by the FDA in November 1999 for use in rheumatoid arthritis. This drug is a synthetic antibody that inhibits the effects of tumor necrosis factor and thus reduces inflammation. It is given intravenously. After the first three doses, maintenance doses are given every eight weeks. Infliximab is associated with many side effects, including nausea, chest pain, fever, cough, facial flushing, headache, itch, indigestion, low blood pressure, and risk of serious infection and lymphomas. This drug should not be taken by anyone who has an infection or who is susceptible to infections.

Drug Alert: Not All Painkillers Are Alike

Some people with rheumatoid arthritis mistakenly believe that any painkiller can be effective. However, painkillers that do not also reduce inflammation can actually cause considerable damage to the joints. If pain is suppressed but inflammation is not, use of the affected joints can trigger release of enzymes that damage ligaments and bone. Drugs such as acetaminophen (Tylenol and others), as well as codeine, Percodan, Darvon, Talwin, and Demerol are effective against pain but do not reduce inflammation. These drugs should not be used by people who have rheumatoid arthritis.

OTHER DRUGS

People who have very severe rheumatoid arthritis may be given immunosuppressant drugs, which suppress the body's overly active immune system. These drugs (cyclosporine [Neoral, Sandimmune], azathioprine [Imuran], cyclophosphamide [Cytoxan], and chlorambucil [Leukeran]) are potentially very toxic. Side effects include gastrointestinal problems, rash, mouth sores, anemia, and other blood disorders.

Use of oral and injected corticosteroids, such as prednisolone and prednisone, can help slow joint destruction and provide rapid control of inflammation and pain. Injections are usually reserved for relief of flare-ups when only one or a few joints are involved. Unfortunately, corticosteroids can cause weight gain, hypertension, acne, excess hair growth, cataracts, glaucoma, dia-

betes, irritability, greater susceptibility to infection, menstrual irregularities, accelerated hardening of the arteries, psychosis, and
insomnia. Long-term use may cause memory loss.

SURGERY

Surgery is sometimes performed in cases of severely affected
joints. The most successful surgeries have been on the knees and
hips and involve either removing the synovium or doing a total
joint replacement. In most individuals who have nearly or completely lost their ability to walk, knee or hip replacement can
make it possible for them to be independent again.

❖ EVALUATION AND TREATMENT OF RHEUMATOID ARTHRITIS: MY APPROACH

The approach to rheumatoid arthritis taken by myself and many
other clinical molecular medicine practitioners is to first conduct
an extensive evaluation of the patient's medical and environmental history, symptoms, and test results (see chapter 2) and then
choose the appropriate evaluation based on those findings. To illustrate that process, we will visit with Lydia, a woman with
rheumatoid arthritis who came to the Edelson Center after having undergone drug treatment unsuccessfully.

Evaluating Lydia

Lydia, a forty-five-year-old clerical assistant, came to me with a
diagnosis of rheumatoid arthritis that had been made one year
earlier. She had been taking various NSAIDs and methotrexate
before coming to see me, and wanted to get off the drugs and find
a permanent solution to her pain and stiffness. "My boss has been
real understanding about my inability to work full-time," she

said. "The company kept me on part-time, but that meant a cut in pay, which has been hard. I can't work much on the computer, and there are lots of other things I can't do, like play on the company bowling team or even open jars. Sometimes I feel so frustrated and helpless."

As we discussed her history, Lydia told me about how during her childhood, her parents used to spray pesticides both in and around their home several times a year, especially on their lawn and shrubbery close to the house. Her father's hobby was restoring antique furniture, so the smell of paint remover, shellac, and other harsh chemicals was constantly in the air at home. In addition, Lydia had worked for a printer for five years, where she was exposed to various printers' chemicals, and she was a smoker.

Her main complaints when she came to me included swollen, painful joints, eczema, allergies, night sweats, fatigue, mastalgia (breast pain), and restless legs syndrome. Considering her history and her symptoms, I decided on the following tests:

• Heavy metal challenge. The results showed significant levels of lead and very high levels of mercury. These two heavy metals cause free-radical damage to the joints and, more importantly, can damage the immune system, creating an "overactivated" one with the ability to react negatively to food, bacteria, and other substances.

• Skin and blood tests for allergies. Revealed severe food allergies. These often contribute to inflammation and pain as well as to malabsorption of nutrients (see amino acid analysis, below).

• CDSA stool study. Showed raised levels of the bacteria *Proteus,* which is often found in people who have rheumatoid arthritis.

• Amino acid analysis. Showed deficiencies, with probable decrease in acid production and malabsorption syndrome. These problems went hand in hand with her severe food allergies.

• DHEA and IgF1 deficiencies. Low levels of DHEA (a hormone) and IgF1 (a protein produced in the liver) are often seen in people who have chronic chemical toxicity and free-radical damage to their organs. These deficiencies are seen in many autoimmune disorders, including rheumatoid arthritis.

• Lipid peroxide levels. Elevated, indicating oxidative stress.

• Antinuclear antibody (ANA) levels. Elevated, as is common in rheumatoid arthritis.

• Rheumatoid factor (RF). Although this was negative, all other test results, and her symptoms, indicated rheumatoid arthritis.

• C-reactive protein. Elevated, as it often is in people who have rheumatoid arthritis.

• DNA injury (8-OHDg). Showed damage to DNA, indicative of oxidative stress and seen in individuals with chemical and/or heavy metal toxicity.

• Tumor necrosis factor. Severely elevated levels, highly indicative of rheumatoid arthritis.

• Natural killer cell activity. Decreased, which indicates a deficiency in cellular immunity (the ability to fight invaders). This activity is often seen in people with chemical and/or heavy metal toxicity.

Treating Rheumatoid Arthritis

Once the joints have been damaged by inflammation, healing becomes much more difficult. That's why early, aggressive treatment is recommended. Conventional treatment of rheumatoid arthritis involves approaches that largely treat symptoms, which means the damage continues or, at best, does not get much worse. Some progress is being made in developing drugs that reduce or halt joint damage, although they can cause significant side effects.

I believe that a much more practical approach to treating rheumatoid arthritis involves impacting the autoimmune process at the cellular level and returning the immune system to a healthy state. In this section we discuss my approach to rheumatoid arthritis, using Lydia's case as an example.

Treating Lydia

As is often the case in rheumatoid arthritis, Lydia had high levels of heavy metals such as mercury and lead, which needed to be removed. She also had poor nutrition—evidenced by her amino acid deficiency, malabsorption, and food allergies—which was contributing to her free-radical activity and fueling her rheumatoid arthritis. The results of the stool sample and levels of ANA, DHEA, IgF1, C-reactive protein, and tumor necrosis factor all indicated the presence of autoimmunity and toxicity. Her lipid peroxide and DNA injury tests confirmed oxidative stress. We began the following treatment:

• Nutritional therapy, including amino acid supplementation to correct her deficiency, and antioxidant therapy, to help fight the free-radical damage and improve the ability of her liver to perform its detoxication function.

• Chelation therapy, using DMPS and DMSA to remove the heavy metals from her body.

• Ozone therapy, which modulates the immune system, improves oxygenation of tissue, and improves antioxidant enzyme activity, all of which work together to help break down toxins.

• High-temperature sauna therapy, to help remove the toxic chemicals from her body.

• Avoidance diet, to eliminate the allergic and intolerance reactions, which were fueling her free-radical and inflammatory processes. Lydia was allergic to corn and wheat and intolerant of dairy products and many other foods.

• EPD, an immunotherapy approach, which helped desensitize Lydia's body to the foods to which she was hypersensitive.

• DMSO, a chemical used to relieve pain caused by inflammation (see box).

• Environmental controls, which meant Lydia had to stop smoking and avoid secondhand smoke. She also installed air purifiers and water purifiers in her home, and was advised to eat whole, organic foods and avoid any foods that had been treated with hormones, antibiotics, or other drugs (found in most meats and dairy products).

• Antibiotics: minocycline (for one year), which appears to block the enzymes that break down cartilage; and clindamycin (for one month). My treatment approach for autoimmune conditions is nearly 100 percent drug-free. However, in some cases a limited course of a few selected drugs may be used. These two antibiotics have proven useful in stopping the progression of rheumatoid arthritis.

DMSO: A Smelly Solution

What if you were offered a treatment that was very effective at relieving arthritic pain and inflammation, that was an antibacterial, antiviral, and antifungal, and that was an antioxidant. And, oh yes, it also makes you emit a strong odor like fish, so strong that your spouse or partner is likely to ask you to sleep in another room. That substance is DMSO, or dimethyl sulfoxide. This chemical has been around for decades and has been used successfully to treat racehorses and athletes to help them with painful, inflamed joints and muscles. DMSO affects altered cellular function and creates changes in protein and water molecules, which results in healed and restored cells. The upshot is that it is useful in the treatment of rheumatoid arthritis, as well as other inflammatory conditions, including multiple sclerosis, lupus, ulcerative colitis, and scleroderma, among others.

My experience with DMSO in patients with rheumatoid arthritis has shown that it can dramatically reduce inflammation and pain. Although it is not a cure, it does allow patients a level of relief they have not been able to reach with other treatments.

As for side effects, it can cause headache when taken in high doses, and at the Edelson Center we do use large doses. The only other downside is the odor, which some patients say is a small price to pay for the return of pain-free mobility.

Although the Food and Drug Administration (FDA) has not approved DMSO for use in arthritis or most other conditions, it has approved its use for interstitial cystitis. This severely painful condition is characterized by inflammation and irritation of the bladder and mostly affects middle-aged women. The FDA approval for cystitis means that doctors may use DMSO at their discretion for other conditions.

After just two to three months, Lydia showed much improvement, especially as her lead and mercury levels dropped dramatically and her tumor necrosis factor levels also declined. Two years after starting therapy, she is doing very well. She has returned to work full-time and is on her company's bowling team.

❖ WHAT YOU CAN DO NOW

• Find a doctor who performs the tests and uses the treatments discussed in this chapter (see chapter 2).

• Make your home environment as toxin-free as possible (see chapter 11 for specific suggestions). I recommend installation of HEPA filters and water filters, and avoidance of all pesticides, insecticides, herbicides, and household cleaning chemicals.

• Switch to a whole foods, organic diet that includes lots of fruits and vegetables and whole grains. You want to avoid hormones, steroids, and food additives, preservatives, and colorings (see chapter 12).

• Ask your doctor to test you for food allergies.

• Take essential fatty acids in the form of organic, unrefined flaxseed oil, 1 to 2 tablespoons daily.

• Use one or more of the herbal chelators (burdock root, dandelion root, lemon balm, milk thistle, uva ursi, yellow dock; at the discretion of your healthcare provider) listed in chapter 11. Always consult with your healthcare provider before using herbs. I do not recommend use of these herbs as the only biodetoxification approach.

• Consider using the nutritional chelators (glutathione, lipoic acid, cysteine, N-acetylcysteine) listed in chapter 11. Always consult with your physician before taking these supplements to determine the proper dosage and which ones are most appropriate for you.

• Take antioxidants and other essential nutrients. You can see a list of the suggested supplements and dosages in chapter 12.

Chapter 7

Crohn's Disease and Ulcerative Colitis

Whaat does it feel like to live with chronic diarrhea? What is it like to always need to be near a bathroom, or to be afraid of having an accident? People who have inflammatory bowel disease—which includes Crohn's disease and ulcerative colitis—can tell you the answers to those questions. And as you can guess, what they have to say is not positive.

In this chapter we discuss these life-altering autoimmune inflammatory bowel conditions and how they affect an estimated one million Americans. More important, you will learn what you can do if you or a loved one are among those afflicted.

❖ INFLAMMATORY BOWEL DISEASE TODAY

Crohn's disease and ulcerative colitis are the two most common types of inflammatory bowel disease (IBD), a general term for inflammatory conditions that damage the digestive tract. (For convenience, when referring to both of these conditions, we use the acronym IBD; when we wish to make a distinction, we use each term separately.) Both of these conditions share many of the same symptoms, although there are some differences, all of which we discuss later in this chapter.

Both diseases typically first affect people between the ages of fifteen and thirty-five. Unlike many other autoimmune disorders, however, Crohn's disease and ulcerative colitis affect men and women equally. Whites have the highest risk of developing these diseases, but people of all ethnic groups can be affected. People of Jewish European ancestry are five to six times more likely to have inflammatory bowel diseases than other whites.

❖ IS INFLAMMATORY BOWEL DISEASE AN AUTOIMMUNE DISORDER?

There is much we still do not understand about these inflammatory bowel diseases. Although we do know that they involve an inflammatory process, no autoantibodies have been definitively identified. One theory that links autoimmunity with IBDs is that some individuals have a genetic susceptibility that allows invading organisms, such as bacteria, viruses, or other environmental factors (chemical toxins and heavy metals), to trigger an abnormal immune response possibly caused by free radicals or by direct effect of the toxic agents. That response includes chronic inflammation of the intestinal tract, the region of the body targeted in the people with this predisposition. Scientists have identified some of the specific types of free radicals responsible for IBD, and they include superoxide ions, hydrogen peroxide, and nitric oxide.

Another immune response seen in people who have IBD is an increase in white blood cells called helper T-cells, which in turn produce damaging proteins called cytokines (see chapter 1). Among these cytokines are tumor necrosis factors, which harm the intestinal tract and also produce more helper T-cells, thus setting up a vicious cycle of damage. So, even though scientists have not identified the exact reason why the immune system launches an attack against the intestinal tract, the fact that it does points to autoimmunity.

❖ COURSE OF THE DISEASE

Like many of the autoimmune diseases, Crohn's disease and ulcerative colitis can run an erratic course. Some people experience months or even years of remission, when they have no symptoms, only to have them appear again suddenly. Others have mild to moderate symptoms on a fairly steady basis, with short remissions. This roller-coaster of symptoms makes it impossible to know whether a treatment has helped or when the disease may flare up, causing people to live with constant uncertainty.

"It's hard for me to plan my wedding," said Brielle, a twenty-four-year-old graduate student who was diagnosed with Crohn's disease at nineteen. At the time she got engaged, she had been in remission for about six months. "Tom and I want to get married in eight months, and we want to go to Europe for our honeymoon, but what if we make big plans and then I have a relapse? That would ruin everything."

Unfortunately, there is no way to predict the rise and fall of the disease. With careful treatment, most people with IBD function well, and death related to Crohn's disease and ulcerative colitis is very low. However, people who have had Crohn's disease of the small intestine for many years are at increased risk of small intestine cancer. A greater risk of colorectal cancer is found among patients with Crohn's disease of the colon and people who have ulcerative colitis.

❖ CAUSES, RISK FACTORS, AND TRIGGERS

Sometimes when scientists are looking for the cause of a disease and they are perplexed, it helps to list the things that *don't* cause the condition. At one time, researchers believed that stress was a cause of Crohn's disease and ulcerative colitis. They no longer think that this is true, yet stress may aggravate symptoms. They also do not believe that these conditions are contagious and are passed along from one person to another, even though one theory holds that a bacterium or virus may be a cause (see "Environmental Factors," below).

As with other autoimmune conditions, we turn to genetics and environmental factors as the causes and triggers of Crohn's disease and ulcerative colitis.

Genetics

Up to 25 percent of people who have Crohn's disease or ulcerative colitis have a parent, sibling, or child who also has an inflammatory bowel disease. The risk is highest if your mother has IBD, followed by a sibling. Fathers pose the least inherited risk to their sons and daughters. It is also common for people who have either of these IBDs to have other autoimmune disorders as well. The fact that Jewish people of European descent are up to six times more likely to have IBD reinforces the strong role of genetics in these diseases.

Environmental Factors

Many scientists believe that an unknown bacterium or virus plays a role in IBD (see "Is Inflammatory Bowel Disease an Autoimmune Disorder?") and that the inflammation is the result of the immune system fighting off the organisms. This theory is supported by the fact that drugs that suppress the immune system (see "Diagnosis and Treatment of Crohn's Disease and Ulcerative Colitis: Conventional Approach," below) have been somewhat effective in some people with Crohn's disease or ulcerative colitis. So far, however, no specific virus or bacterium has been definitively identified as the culprit.

COULD IT BE A MYCOBACTERIUM?

One bacterium in particular has attracted some attention. Some researchers suggest that *Mycobacterium avium-paratuberculosis* (MAP, found in milk) is linked with Crohn's disease. Professor John-Hermon Taylor, an expert on Crohn's disease and chairman of the Department of Surgery at St. George's Hospital Medical School in London, has said that "if there was no MAP, though difficult to detect and destroy, there would be no Crohn's." But there is MAP: between 20 and 40 percent of U.S. dairy herds are infected with the bacteria. MAP is transmitted inside pus, and American milk consumers are exposed to a great deal of pus: by U.S. federal law, grade A milk is allowed to contain more than a drop of pus per glass of milk.

Several studies, including those conducted by Dr. Taylor, have linked MAP with Crohn's disease. In one study, researchers found MAP in 65 percent of Crohn's patients, compared with only 12.5 percent of controls. Their work was later replicated by six other independent research groups. The threat of MAP and Crohn's disease has so concerned the government of the United Kingdom that in December 2001, lawmakers adopted comprehensive strategies to prevent human exposure to the organism by eliminating it from retail milk.

Yet in the United States there continues to be denial of a problem by the dairy industry and the Department of Agriculture. At this time, it is unknown what percentage of cases of Crohn's disease may be caused by MAP.

COULD IT BE DIET?

Another aspect of diet also appears to play a significant role in IBD. Scientists have noted that while IBD appears primarily among people who eat a diet high in animal protein, refined foods, fat, and sugar, it is virtually unknown among cultures where people consume a simple diet of whole grains, legumes, fruits, and vegetables. Again, we can't say for certain that diet causes IBD, but it seems hard to deny that it has a significant impact and could trigger onset.

Yet another theory links antibiotics with Crohn's disease. One argument for this is that the dramatic rise in the incidence of the disease has paralleled the tremendous increase in the use of antibiotics. This includes antibiotics given for medical conditions as well as people's exposure to antibiotics in meat and dairy products. It is known that antibiotics can destroy the good bacteria in the intestinal tract, making the bowel susceptible to damage and disease.

We must also consider food sensitivities. In people who have food sensitivities, the intestinal lining reacts to certain foods, which can definitely worsen inflammatory bowel disease. This reaction can lead to more inflammation and free-radical production. It is classic among people with inflammatory bowel disease that when you remove the foods to which they are allergic or sensitive, their symptoms decrease.

IBD: What's Going On in There?

To understand IBD, it helps to know about the gastrointestinal (GI) tract. The upper part of the GI tract includes the mouth, esophagus, stomach, duodenum, liver, spleen, and pancreas. The lower portion consists of the intestine, which is composed of two parts: the small intestine (about six meters long) and the large intestine, or colon (about two meters). The small intestine has two main parts: the jejunum (upper part) and the ileum (lower part). The large intestine consists of the cecum, ascending colon, transverse colon, descending colon, sigmoid colon, and rectum. Crohn's disease can affect any part of the GI tract, from the mouth to the rectum. Ulcerative colitis affects the colon and rectum only.

The primary task of the small intestine is to digest and absorb dietary nutrients; the colon mainly absorbs water and moves along stool. Both the small and large intestines work together with the liver and pancreas to break down complex foods and to extract the nutrients they need to pass along to the bloodstream.

The intestines have a thin underlying layer called the submucosa, where the blood vessels and lymph channels run. Covering the submucosa is a lining called the mucosa. In Crohn's disease, both the mucosa and submucosa are affected; in ulcerative colitis, only the mucosa is inflamed.

❖ SIGNS AND SYMPTOMS

Crohn's disease and ulcerative colitis have many similar and a few differing signs and symptoms. Perhaps the biggest difference between the two inflammatory bowel diseases is that Crohn's disease can affect any part of the digestive tract. That means inflammation, ulcers, and fistulas (see below) can appear in the mouth, stomach, large intestine, or points in between. In fact, affected or diseased sections along the gastrointestinal tract may be separated by normal segments, a condition that is referred to as "skip lesions." The presence of skip lesions can make it more difficult for doctors to diagnose the disease.

In ulcerative colitis, inflammation is typically limited to the rectum and colon, and fistulas are not involved. Here are other similarities and differences between these two diseases.

Crohn's Disease

Crohn's disease (also known as regional enteritis, granulomatous colitis, or ileocolitis) was first described in 1932 by Burrill B. Crohn, M.D., and his associates. They explained that it was an inflammatory reaction of the bowel that usually affected the ileum, the colon, or other parts of the gastrointestinal tract. Here are the signs and symptoms associated with the disease. They may be mild to severe, and they can change in intensity from day to day.

• **Diarrhea.** Loose, watery bowel movements are probably secondary to inflammation of the colon and a decrease in its ability to absorb water. The severity of the diarrhea can range from four or fewer watery or loose bowel movements daily (mild Crohn's disease) to more than six movements daily (severe disease).

• **Bleeding.** Blood may be mixed in with stool or be eliminated along with stool. Bleeding may occur as food waste passes through the inflamed intestinal system and irritates the intestinal walls, or the tissue may bleed on its own.

• **Ulcers.** Open sores (ulcers) can develop anywhere along the digestive tract, although in Crohn's disease they usually occur in the lower small intestine, colon, or rectum.

• **Weight loss and fatigue.** These symptoms can occur if the small intestine is inflamed, thus preventing absorption of nutrients. Fatigue can also result from blood loss and poor nutrient absorption. Malabsorption of nutrients can be a real problem for young people who have Crohn's disease, because it can stunt their growth. Approximately 30 percent of people with IBD are ages ten through nineteen, the growth years.

• **Fistulas.** Imagine a tunnel that connects point A with point B, and you'll have an idea of what a fistula is. A fistula begins as an ulcer that deepens and burrows to form a connection between internal organs, between two points within the same organ, or between an organ and the skin. In Crohn's disease, fistulas can develop between the small intestine and colon, which allows food particles to skip absorption in the small intestine and move on directly to the colon. Fistulas can also become infected.

• **Vomiting and cramping.** Chronic inflammation of the intestinal walls can cause scar tissue to form, which gradually makes the intestinal passageway more narrow. This can lead to cramping and vomiting.

• **Complications.** The most common complication is blockage of the intestine, which can happen when the intestinal walls thicken because of inflammation, scar tissue, and ulcers. Other complications include infected fistulas, which can require surgery in some cases; nutritional deficiencies, which can result from poor absorption (malabsorption) or inadequate nutritional intake; arthritis; rashes or sores; anal skin tags (soft lesions); kidney stones; and gallstones.

Ulcerative Colitis

People who have ulcerative colitis can expect the same symptoms as those in Crohn's disease, with a few modifications. In ulcerative colitis, blood in the stool is very common, along with pus or mucus from the intestinal lining. Complications of ulcerative colitis are generally the same as those in Crohn's disease, except liver disease is seen instead of kidney stones, gallstones, or anal skin tags, and fistulas are not present. Another complication seen in ulcerative colitis is toxic megacolon, which occurs in 2 to 6 percent of patients. Toxic megacolon develops when the colon becomes inflamed and unable to eliminate stool or gas. This causes the colon to enlarge (megacolon) and results in abdominal swelling and pain, fever, weakness, and feeling disoriented. If not treated, the colon can rupture and leak bacteria into the abdominal area, leading to serious infection.

❖ DIAGNOSIS AND TREATMENT OF CROHN'S DISEASE AND ULCERATIVE COLITIS: CONVENTIONAL APPROACH

Both Crohn's disease and ulcerative colitis can be difficult to diagnose because their symptoms are similar not only to each other but also to other intestinal disorders, such as irritable bowel syndrome. Also, in women, the pain and inflammation associated with Crohn's disease are similar to those caused by pelvic inflammatory disease, ectopic pregnancy, and ovarian tumors and cysts. So, like many other autoimmune diseases, IBDs are identified after all other probable causes are ruled out.

Making a Diagnosis

The first step is to take a thorough history and evaluation of the patient, followed by tests that can help doctors reach a diagnosis of Crohn's disease or ulcerative colitis. Here are the main tools doctors use to reach a diagnosis.

- **Sedimentation rate.** Abnormal levels on this blood test indicate inflammation and IBD.
- **Complete blood count (CBC).** Among other things, this test may be done to check for anemia, which suggests bleeding in the intestines. Doctors also look for a high white blood cell count, which indicates inflammation.
- **C-reactive protein.** High levels of this substance indicate systemic inflammation.
- **Stool test.** This is done to see if there is bleeding or infection in the intestinal tract.
- **Barium enema.** This test, which involves a thick, chalky liquid (barium sulfate) given in an enema, allows doctors to visualize the colon and rectum.
- **Upper GI series.** In this test, you drink a chalky barium solution that coats the lining of the esophagus, stomach, duodenum, and small intestine. Various monitoring devices are used to track the progress of the barium, which helps doctors identify any inflammation or other abnormalities in the upper gastrointestinal and small bowel follow-through procedure.
- **Colonoscopy.** A long (3- to 4-foot), flexible tube called an endoscope is inserted into the anus and up through the large intestine. The endoscope is linked with a computer and monitor, which allow the doctor to detect bleeding and inflammation. A tissue biopsy may be taken from the intestinal lining during the colonoscopy.
- **Sigmoidoscopy.** A short (14- to 24-inch) instrument is in-

serted into the lower bowel to view the colon lining for inflammation and abnormalities, or to take samples. This is typically used to both diagnose and monitor ulcerative colitis.

Treatment

Treatment of IBD focuses on controlling inflammation and relieving symptoms such as pain, bleeding, and diarrhea. The actual treatments chosen depend on the location of the abnormalities, the presence of complications, whether past treatments have failed, and the severity of the disease. Drugs and surgery, as needed, are used to achieve these goals.

Drug Therapy

Drugs in several different categories are used to treat IBD, and many people take more than one drug at a time. Here are the most common ones doctors prescribe:

• **Anti-inflammatory drugs.** These are usually the first drugs prescribed to people who have IBD. Several different ones are available.

➤ Sulfasalazine (Azulfidine) has been available for mild to moderate IBD since the 1940s. People with mild to moderate Crohn's disease or ulcerative colitis can benefit the most from this drug. It can cause loss of appetite, nausea, vomiting, diarrhea, heartburn, rash, and headache.

➤ Mesalamine (Asacol, Pentasa, Rowasa) is often taken by people who cannot tolerate sulfasalazine, and it causes fewer side effects than that drug. When mesalamine is used in an enema, it can relieve symptoms in more than 80 percent of people who have ulcerative colitis of the lower colon and rectum. Olsalazine (Dipentum), another anti-inflammatory drug, is similar to mesalamine.

➤ Corticosteroids (e.g., prednisone, hydrocortisone) are another type of anti-inflammatory drug used to treat IBD, but they are usually reserved for moderate to severe disease that does not respond to other treatment. Corticosteroids are associated with many side effects, including high blood pressure, puffy face, acne, night sweats, insomnia, and hyperactivity.

• **Immunosuppressants.** These drugs reduce inflammation by suppressing the immune system's ability to release the chemicals that are causing the inflammation.

➤ The ones most commonly prescribed are azathioprine (Imuran) and 6-mercaptopurine (6-MP). It can take from three to six months for these drugs to relieve symptoms, including healing of fistulas. However, they can reduce a person's resistance to infection as well as cause nausea, vomiting, and diarrhea. Allergy and pancreatitis (inflamed pancreas) can also be a problem.

➤ The newest addition to this category for treatment of IBD is infliximab (Remicade), which is for people with moderate to severe Crohn's disease. It works by neutralizing tumor necrosis factor, a substance that causes inflammation. Although it has shown much promise, its benefits appear to decrease over time, and more long-term studies are needed. This drug greatly increases a person's risk of infection (in about one-third of users).

➤ People who don't respond to or who can't tolerate other medications may be given methotrexate or cyclosporine. Methotrexate can cause nausea in the short run, and liver problems with long-term use. Cyclosporine is usually best for people with Crohn's disease who have fistulas or for severe ulcerative colitis. Long-term use can produce excessive hair growth, seizures, high blood pressure, liver and kidney damage, and numbness of the hands.

• **Antibiotics.** These are generally given to people with Crohn's disease to help heal fistulas and ulcers. Sometimes they can cause remission of symptoms.

➤ Metronidazole (Flagyl) is one of the more commonly prescribed antibiotics for Crohn's disease, but it can cause many serious side effects. About one-third of people who take metronidazole experience tingling and numbness in the hands and feet, pain, and muscle weakness. Other adverse reactions include headache, nausea, yeast infection, and loss of appetite.

➤ Ciprofloxacin (Cipro) is also commonly used. About half of patients who take this antibiotic can expect some relief. Side effects include hypersensitivity to light and, in children, stunting of growth.

• **Other medications.** Medications often given to relieve symptoms include antidiarrheals (Metamucil, Citrucel, Imodium), pain relievers (Tylenol), and iron supplements for those who have anemia from bleeding.

Lifestyle Changes

Not all doctors agree that lifestyle changes can make a significant difference in how people live with IBD, so some patients don't get the essential dietary and stress management information they need to help them heal. The suggestions given here are offered by some conventional physicians who realize their value in managing symptoms and healing the gastrointestinal tract. I, however, use a more aggressive lifestyle-change approach (see "Treating Leonard," below, for more information).

• Limit dairy products. Some people with Crohn's disease experience a great improvement in gastrointestinal symptoms when they reduce (or even better, eliminate) dairy products from their diet. That's because IBD patients have food allergies that may be causing a worsening of their condition. Although there are many soy- and rice-based products that you can substitute for dairy foods, some people are sensitive or allergic to them as well. I believe all patients should be aggressively tested (using both skin and blood tests) for allergies and sensitivities to dairy as well as other types of foods as part of their initial evaluation.

• Experiment with high-fiber foods. Although fruits, grains, and vegetables are excellent sources of many nutrients, most of them also supply fiber. For some people with IBD, fiber can worsen diarrhea and gas. Individuals with IBD need to discuss their dietary needs with a clinical molecular medicine physician, who can help them not only select foods they can eat but also ensure they will get all the nutrients they need.

• Take a multivitamin-mineral supplement. I personally believe nutritional supplementation is critical, given that IBD interferes with absorption of nutrients. Supplementation should be supervised by your doctor to make sure you get the correct dosages for your personal needs, especially if you are taking medications that can hinder the absorption of nutrients.

• Reduce fat intake. If you have severe Crohn's disease of the small intestine, you won't be able to absorb fat properly. Too much fat in your diet will likely worsen diarrhea.

• Drink at least eight glasses of water daily. Diarrhea depletes the body of essential water and minerals, so rehydration is important. Also, avoid beverages that promote urine loss, such as those containing caffeine and alcohol.

• Manage and reduce stress. Stress can worsen IBD symptoms and provoke flare-ups. This occurs because during stressful times, more stomach acid is produced and more free radicals are created. The result is that the passage of waste through the intestines is speeded up. Routine exercise, deep breathing, meditation, yoga, relaxation exercises, and other forms of stress reduction are recommended daily.

Surgery

Up to 20 percent of people with ulcerative colitis and 70 percent of those with Crohn's disease do not respond to drug treatment and lifestyle changes and need surgery. Among people with Crohn's disease, surgery is done to remove blockages, abscesses, or perforations, or to relieve symptoms, including bleeding. A major problem with surgery for Crohn's disease is that the disease usually recurs after surgery, which leads 75 percent of patients to another surgical procedure. Some people who have Crohn's disease in the large intestine undergo a colectomy, in which the entire colon is removed. They leave the operating room with an opening in their abdomen called a stoma, where waste can leave the body and collect in a pouch worn over the opening. Many colectomy patients go on to live active lives.

❖ EVALUATION AND TREATMENT OF INFLAMMATORY BOWEL DISEASE: MY APPROACH

Perhaps even more than with other autoimmune diseases, the evaluation and treatment of Crohn's disease and ulcerative colitis require much attention to nutrition and reestablishing gastrointestinal health, because the primary target of self-attack is the GI tract. Because nutrition is an area with which most doctors are not familiar, I find that many patients with IBD who come to me have not received adequate guidance on dietary changes and nutritional supplementation, which have a dramatic impact on intestinal health. So along with removing metals and chemical toxins from the body, I believe that people with IBD need to learn which foods may be acting as toxins in their body and eliminate them from their diet, while adding healthy foods and supplements that will promote healing. After a few months of treatment, patients go into remission.

Evaluating Leonard

Crohn's disease had already affected seven of Leonard's twenty-one years of life, and he was not looking forward to living the rest of his life with the disease. Leonard came to the Edelson Center after having gone through years of treatment with traditional drugs, including steroids. "When my last doctor recommended chemotherapy, I said no way," Leonard explained as we discussed his history. "There's got to be a better way to treat this disease."

Leonard had the typical symptoms of Crohn's disease (diarrhea, flatulence, stomach cramps, mucus in stool), along with joint pain. His physical examination and environmental history didn't reveal anything unusual (except for four amalgams), but a discussion of his dietary habits revealed that he was definitely on the wrong track. Although Leonard's other doctors had given him a list of foods to avoid, no concerted effort had been made to follow up with his eating habits or to help him with alternative food choices.

Dietary choices are critical in people who have IBD, yet many doctors are reluctant to emphasize that changes be made.

As a teenager having to cope with peer pressure as well as the restrictions imposed by his autoimmune condition, Leonard was still eating foods that were irritating his GI tract, as he had never undergone any skin or blood tests to identify his food sensitivities or allergies. We proceeded with several lab tests, and here is what we found:

- Heavy metal challenge showed slightly elevated levels of mercury and lead.
- Stool studies showed elevated levels of the bacteria klebsiella, which is often seen in people who have Crohn's disease.
- Intestinal permeability indicated malabsorption (poor absorption of nutrients), common among people who have Crohn's disease.
- Antinuclear antibody (ANA) test was positive.
- Complete blood count (CBC) showed iron-deficiency anemia, common among people who have IBD.
- Immune complex test was positive, a common finding in autoimmunity.
- There was candida in blood with signs of immune complex.
- There was a decrease in pancreatic function, with low levels of chymotrypsin, an enzyme that helps with the breakdown of carbohydrates, fats, and protein.

Treating Leonard

Leonard had the classic signs and symptoms of Crohn's disease, as well as a digestive system that was in dire need of nutritional assistance. Not only was he failing to get the nutrients he needed from his food, but his pancreas was not properly breaking down his food. For Leonard, the following treatment program was established:

• Dietary changes. After skin and blood testing revealed that Leonard was allergic or sensitive to a variety of foods, including dairy, citrus, and wheat, he was able to make the appropriate changes in his diet. He was introduced to calcium- and protein-enriched soy milk and rice milk products and rice and oat flours instead of wheat. Once he substituted these foods and experienced a dramatic improvement in his symptoms, he was willing to make the dietary changes permanent.

• Nutritional therapy. Inflammatory bowel diseases interfere with the absorption of nutrients, but starting an individual on an aggressive oral supplementation program can be ineffective. So our first step with Leonard was to give him an intravenous "cocktail" of antioxidants, amino acids, B vitamins, glutamine, and a mixture of minerals several times a week until his intestinal tract began to heal. Then he was prescribed a high-potency multivitamin-mineral along with additional antioxidants (vitamins C and E, and selenium) and zinc, as he was especially deficient in these nutrients. This type of deficiency is common in people with IBD. Iron supplements were also given to treat his anemia, as well as a calcium/magnesium supplement to ensure he was getting an adequate amount after eliminating dairy products.

• His intestinal bacterial overgrowth of candida was treated aggressively with nystatin and grapefruit seed extract, as Leonard had a severe case. He received:

➤ Itraconazole (Sporanox), an antifungal taken in capsule form.
➤ Neomycin, an antibiotic for the bacterial overgrowth.
➤ The herb aloe vera, which has anti-inflammatory properties and contains mucopolysaccharides, which aid in absorption of nutrients.

➤ Glutamine, which helps improve absorption of nutrients and is also a precursor for the potent antioxidant glutathione.

➤ Leonard was also given a pectin supplement. Pectin helps promote the growth of good bacteria without producing excess stool.

• Ozone therapy. Leonard underwent both rectal and intravenous ozone treatments, which reduce inflammation and improve functioning of the immune system, in turn helping it destroy fungi, bacteria, and viruses, and helping eliminate toxins in the body, among other benefits. Leonard began with three treatments per week for two weeks, and then gradually received fewer and less frequent treatments until he was getting one treatment every other week.

• Chelation therapy. Leonard underwent treatment with DMSA to eliminate the mercury and lead in his system. These heavy metals promote the formation of free radicals, which damage the gastrointestinal tract in IBD.

❖ WHAT YOU CAN DO NOW

• Avoid tap water, foods with preservatives, and nonorganic foods. Also avoid sugary foods. Americans eat a great deal of sugar and foods that have been denatured (stripped of their nutrients), such as white rice, white flour, and all the products made with these ingredients. These food particles ferment in the digestive tract and produce gas rather than being properly and efficiently broken down to be used by the body. Sugary foods are also fuel for candida infections in the intestinal tract. A return to whole, natural (and organic) foods is recommended.

• Ask your doctor to test you for food allergies.

• Many people with IBD take steroids, which can severely deplete levels of the adrenal hormone DHEA. This hormone improves the immune system's ability to fight infections, and so some patients with IBD can benefit from DHEA supplementation. The supplement should only be taken under a doctor's supervision.

• Herbal remedies for IBD include the use of slippery elm and comfrey, which have a soothing effect similar to that of aloe vera; cayenne, which reduces inflammation; and licorice, which has a natural steroidlike effect and helps reduce inflammation. Consult a doctor knowledgeable about herbs before using these products.

• Do not use nonsteroidal anti-inflammatory drugs (NSAIDs), which include aspirin and ibuprofen. They can trigger IBD symptoms and, in one study, were found to double the risk for emergency treatment of GI problems in people who have colitis.

• Find a doctor who performs the tests and uses the treatments discussed in this chapter (see chapter 2).

• Make your home environment as toxin-free as possible (see chapter 11 for specific suggestions). I recommend installation of HEPA filters and water filters, and avoidance of all pesticides, insecticides, herbicides, and household cleaning chemicals.

• Use one or more of the herbal chelators (burdock root, dandelion root, lemon balm, milk thistle, uva ursi, yellow dock; at the discretion of your healthcare provider) listed in chapter 11. Always consult with your healthcare provider before using herbs. I do not recommend use of these herbs as the only biodetoxification approach.

• Consider using the nutritional chelators (glutathione, lipoic acid, cysteine, N-acetylcysteine) listed in chapter 11. Always consult with your physician before taking these supplements to determine the proper dosage and which ones are most appropriate for you.

• Take antioxidants and other essential nutrients. You can see a list of the suggested supplements and dosages in chapter 12.

Chapter 8

Multiple Sclerosis

In 1421, Jan van Bieren, Count of Holland, described what is believed to be the first documented account of multiple sclerosis. The patient, known only as "Lidwina," had developed weakness in her legs and severe facial pain at age fifteen after falling while ice-skating. Within a few years of her fall her leg weakness had progressed until she could no longer walk, and she was intermittently blind in one eye.

It wasn't until the mid-1800s, however, that a scientific description of multiple sclerosis was proposed. Jean-Martin Charcot (1825–1893) worked in a Paris medical facility and examined thousands of patients. He correlated various signs and symptoms he observed in patients with what he saw at autopsies—scarring of the nerves—and described a condition he called *la sclérose en plaques*. Charcot's work led the way for more research into this autoimmune disease that attacks the nervous system.

❖ MULTIPLE SCLEROSIS TODAY

Nearly six centuries have passed since multiple sclerosis (MS) is believed to have been identified, and our knowledge of the condition has improved. Yet what happens to the bodies of the more than 350,000 people in the United States or the estimated one million people worldwide who have been diagnosed with multiple sclerosis is still not well understood. One thing we do know: in the United States, the estimated annual medical, economic, and social costs of MS exceed $2.5 billion. And here's what else we know.

❖ A MATTER OF COMMUNICATION

The body system affected in multiple sclerosis is the central nervous system, which is composed of the brain and spinal cord. The brain consists of billions of nerve cells, or neurons, that are constantly sending electrical messages among themselves. These messages travel along a part of the neuron called the axon and go from the brain and down to the nerves in the spinal cord, as well as up from the spinal-cord nerves back to the brain. Like an incredibly complex telephone system, the transmission of all these signals makes it possible for us to think, move, and feel.

Just as telephone wires are wrapped in insulation to protect the transmitting wires inside, axons are covered in a protective protein coating called myelin. In people with MS, the myelin gets damaged or the axon itself is destroyed, which makes it difficult or impossible for the messages to get through. The brain may be saying "pick up the pencil with your right hand," but the signal gets distorted and the individual either fails to pick up the pencil or does so after some difficulty.

❖ WHY MULTIPLE SCLEROSIS IS AN AUTOIMMUNE DISEASE

For reasons we don't fully understand, the T-lymphocytes, or T-cells, in some people migrate to the nervous system and eyes and, along with macrophages, begin to attack the myelin. The T-cells then produce cytokines, which send out messages to other immune cells to join in the attack. When the attack intensifies, inflammation and scars ("sclerosis" means scarring) result.

The destruction of myelin, called demyelination, seems to be arbitrary and can vary in location and intensity within the same person. The attacks usually continue for the rest of the individual's life.

❖ COURSE OF THE DISEASE

"Unpredictable" is the best word to describe the course of this disease. A main characteristic of multiple sclerosis is the continual loss of brain tissue, even in very early stages of the disease when symptoms are generally mild. Some people get one or two symptoms that stay mild or moderate and then do not get another symptom for months or years. Other individuals get a few symptoms that immediately become worse, and then acquire new ones within a few weeks or months. Heat in the form of hot weather, a hot bath or shower, or a fever can intensify symptoms for many people. Recovery periods cannot be predicted, nor can relapses. Relapses can happen spontaneously or be triggered by an illness, such as a cold or flu.

Symptoms vary a great deal between people with MS, which makes it difficult to create a typical case. We do know that in about 90 percent of all cases, symptoms first appear between the ages of twenty and forty. The first attack may show up as a numbness in the arms or legs that lasts for a few weeks, or vision may be blurred or lost in one eye for a similar amount of time. Some people go to a doctor, who typically finds nothing wrong, while others do nothing and let the symptoms pass, which they will do.

A second and subsequent attacks may occur within weeks, months, or years; there is no way to tell when they will happen. Each attack may involve the same or different symptoms, but recovery from them is usually not complete. Thus an attack of weakness in the legs that makes it impossible to walk without a cane will likely gradually improve until use of a cane is only necessary occasionally. This phase is called the relapsing-remitting (recovery) phase—a time when symptoms come and go, sometimes leaving some residual damage—and this cycle can repeat itself for many years. In between attacks, the damage continues. Over time, the recovery periods tend to be less and less complete. Whether any permanent disability results depends on the extent of damage to the nerves in any given area of the body.

The next phase is the secondary progressive phase, in which individuals usually do not experience recovery periods and so, steadily, although in many cases very slowly, decline. Fortunately, most people who have multiple sclerosis never reach this stage. In fact, most people who have MS live a fairly normal life span.

❖ CAUSES, TRIGGERS, AND RISK FACTORS

Although researchers have not discovered exactly what causes multiple sclerosis, it appears to be a combination of two general factors: genetics and environmental triggers. Although there's nothing you can do about the genes you're born with, there's plenty you can do about environmental factors, which are believed to trigger the disease in susceptible individuals. Fortunately, this fact is helpful when it comes to treatment. First, however, let's look at the two categories of causes

Genetics

• Gender. About twice as many women as men get the disease. Symptoms usually first appear between the ages of twenty and forty years.

• Race. Differences in occurrence of the disease among different races suggest that genetics plays a significant role in who will react to environmental triggers and who will not. Multiple sclerosis is much more common among white people, especially those who live in northern Europe or who are of northern European descent, as are many people who now live in the United States, Canada, and Australia. Yet the disease is rarely seen in whites in South Africa. It is also rare among Asians, blacks, and Native Americans.

• Family history. For people living in North America or northern Europe, the general risk of getting multiple sclerosis is 1 in 1,000, or 0.1 percent. If your mother or sister has MS, your risk of getting the disease is about 3 percent. If your fraternal twin has MS, your risk is still 3 percent, but if your identical twin has the disease, your risk is 30 percent. A significant finding reported in the December 2000 issue of *Annals of Neurology* shows that the offspring of parents who both have MS have about a 33 percent chance of getting the disease. Because the risk of getting the disease in such cases is not 100 percent, this finding supports the idea that genetics is a factor, but not the only one, in determining who will get this disease. This is where environmental factors come in.

Environmental Factors

• Cooler locations. One of the most unusual things about MS is that it is more common in cooler latitudes. Scientists have defined "cooler latitudes" as being above 40 degrees north (from Boulder, Colorado, or Columbus, Ohio, north) and below 40 degrees south (southern Australia, New Zealand, southern Chile, Argentina). This doesn't mean that people who live south of Boulder or Columbus don't get MS; the disease is just much more prevalent at higher latitudes. MS develops in 1 out of every 2,000 people who grow up at higher latitudes, compared with 1 out of every 10,000 born in lower latitudes. People who grow up near the equator rarely get the disease. Another curious finding is that where a person spent the first decade of life seems to be the deciding factor as to whether he or she will get MS. So far, no one has identified why any of this is true.

• Contagious infection. Some doctors believe a viral or bacterial infection triggers MS in a genetically susceptible person. But the authors of the study published in December 2000 of *Annals of Neurology* say that based on their research, which included more than 13,000 patients with MS, a viral or bacterial infection is unlikely to cause the disease. Only 23 of the patients had a significant other who also had MS, which is a rate of less than 0.2 percent, similar to that found in the general population.

• Internal toxins. Some scientists have proposed that internal toxins—those produced by bacteria and fungi that dwell in the gastrointestinal tract, including *Candida albicans,* a common yeast—can cause MS symptoms.

• Environmental toxins. One prominent theory suggests that heavy metals, such as mercury, aluminum, and lead, replace the normal, balanced molecules in the myelin sheaths, which leads to an increase in free radicals. The damage the free radicals cause results in multiple sclerosis. Because the immune system now recognizes this newly damaged tissue as foreign, it attacks, resulting in an autoimmune process and further damage to the body.

Environmental Toxin Theory

Although we are exposed to dozens of toxic elements in our environment, two of the most common ones are lead and mercury. Both substances are easily inhaled or ingested into the body and absorbed into the bloodstream, where they can be carried over the blood-brain barrier. The blood-brain barrier is a sophisticated roadblock, designed to protect the brain—and thus the very fragile central nervous system—from intruders that can cause damage. Unfortunately, toxins like mercury and lead outsmart the barrier, and once they reach the nervous system, they can stimulate free-radical damage throughout it.

Mercury toxicity can cause a wide variety of health problems, including fatigue, blurred vision, hearing loss, unsteady gait (ataxia), creeping and tingling sensations on the skin (paresthesias), malaise (tiredness), impaired smell or taste, insomnia, loss of appetite, irritability, depression, short-term memory loss, tremors, muscle weakness in the limbs, headache, and cerebral palsy. If you have multiple sclerosis, you probably recognize this list immediately: all of the symptoms, with the exception of the last one, are symptoms of the disease (see "Signs and Symptoms," below).

Mercury and lead are not the only environmental factors that can interrupt the body's normal metabolic processes and damage the myelin sheath of nerves, says Gary Oberg, M.D., past president of the American Academy of Environmental Medicine. He, as well as myself and other doctors who practice environmental medicine, believes that substances such as carbon monoxide, diesel fumes, solvents, aerosol sprays, foam and chipboard in furniture and carpets, and chemicals in food and tap water can produce or aggravate symptoms of MS. Although these substances are toxic for everyone, they may initiate an autoimmune reaction in susceptible individuals.

❖ SIGNS AND SYMPTOMS

One of the things that makes it so difficult to diagnose multiple sclerosis is that it is associated with a great many signs and symptoms. Add to that fact the idea that the immune system seems to arbitrarily choose which nerves to damage and that the areas damaged and the extent to which they are damaged differ for each person who has MS, and it becomes obvious that no two people with the disease have the same symptoms.

Pinpointing the Damage

Which signs and symptoms affect any given person depends on where in the body the myelin is damaged. For example, if the cerebellum and cerebrum in the brain are damaged, there are likely to be problems with balance, speech, coordination, and tremors. If motor nerves are attacked, symptoms will probably include bowel and bladder problems, spasticity paralysis, difficulties with vision, and muscle weakness. Damage to sensory nerves usually results in numbness, tingling, and changes in sensation.

Caroline is an example of someone who has the latter type of damage. She was diagnosed with multiple sclerosis in 2000 at the age of twenty-eight, and she came to see me a year later to "understand the biology of my illness." She was in the early stages of the disease, and her main complaints were a tingling in her extremities and foot drop (when the muscles on the top part of the ankle weaken, preventing people from holding the foot level and thus causing the toes to catch on the ground or floor, leading to falls). Lab test results indicated that her myelin damage was likely due, at least in part, to toxic levels of DDE and organophosphorus pesticides and elevated levels of mercury (she had seventeen amalgams) and lead, among other findings.

The primary complaints of another patient, Olivia, pointed to motor nerve damage. She was diagnosed with multiple sclerosis at twenty-one, shortly after she experienced intermittent blurring and blindness in one eye. This was followed by muscle weakness in her legs, which caused her to collapse at times. Among the findings on her evaluation were very high levels of mercury and lead.

FATIGUE

Fatigue is the most common symptom of MS, occurring in about 78 percent of people with the disease. It usually strikes hardest in late afternoon, although many people experience bouts of it throughout the day.

That is true for Barbara, whose motto is "early to bed, late to rise, and naps in between." That's how this twenty-nine-year-old graphic artist describes her formula for dealing with the overwhelming fatigue that plagues her every day. For some people with MS, the fatigue makes it impossible for them to hold down a full-time job or class schedule or to leave the house for more than a few hours at a time. Barbara considers herself to be lucky because she does freelance work out of her home. After eating breakfast, she can usually work for an hour or two before she needs a nap. Then she can often make it through lunch until about three o'clock before she needs to lie down again. It's rare for her to stay awake past eight o'clock, so "I'm not much fun on a date," she says, and the truth is, she rarely has the strength to go out. Sometimes an extra-long nap in the afternoon gives her the strength to stay up later for special occasions.

DEPRESSION

One symptom that affects about 50 percent of people with MS and that is not a direct result of myelin damage is depression. About 12 percent of people with MS are severely depressed, compared with 5 percent of the general population. Those who have the most disabilities are the most likely to be depressed. One reason the depression rate is high among people with MS is that the disease typically affects young people who are faced with living the rest of their lives with the condition. That prospect is likely the reason suicide is three to ten times more common among people with MS than in the general population. One of the truly gratifying parts of my work is that I have treated individuals who have MS and have seen them improve significantly; that improvement has made their lives worth living.

SENSORY COMPLAINTS: BURNING, TINGLING, NUMBNESS

Up to 55 percent of patients experience crawling sensations, numbness, tingling, or burning in their limbs or trunk area. These sensory complaints are often among the first symptoms of the disease. Some people describe the feeling as "worms wiggling in my feet" or "ants crawling under my skin."

PAIN

Although people with MS have the same pains that the general population feels, such as headache and temporary muscle pain, 20 to 50 percent of them experience types of pain that are the result of short-circuit problems that occur between the neurons in the brain and the spinal cord. One type is an excruciating, stabbing pain in the face known as trigeminal neuralgia, which usually lasts from seconds to several minutes. The pain can recur over months but eventually usually disappears on its own.

Another type of pain is called Lhermitte's sign. The first time Juan felt this unusual pain, he was frightened. "All I did was turn my head and look down, and this pain shot down my spine and into my legs," he said. "I didn't know what was happening." Lhermitte's sign is brief and more distressful than discomforting. It often occurs early in the disease course.

WEAKNESS

This symptom is very common and can be debilitating, especially in those who are also suffering with spasticity or balance problems. Treatment depends on the cause of the weakness: muscle fatigue, lack of use of the muscle, or a nerve transmission problem. A tired muscle can be rested, one that has not been used can be exercised, but if the weakness is caused by a communication problem in the nerves, there is no effective treatment at present.

TREMORS

Trembling or shaking of an arm or leg or occasionally the head, lips, tongue, or jaw affects up to 50 percent of people who have MS. Because tremors can come and go unexpectedly, they are often associated with balance and coordination problems when they affect the limbs. The most common type of tremor associated with MS is intentional tremor, which results when demyelination occurs in the cerebellum, the part of the brain responsible for balance and muscle coordination.

SPASTICITY

In normal movement, two opposing groups of muscles work together: one relaxes while the other contracts. In people who have MS, opposing muscle groups sometimes contract simultaneously, resulting in spasticity, or constant muscle stiffness. Unfortunately, spasticity most often affects the larger muscles, like those in the calf, thigh, upper arm, and forearm, which can make normal activities like walking, eating, getting dressed, and lifting difficult.

BLADDER AND BOWEL PROBLEMS

Normal emptying of the bladder depends on clear communication between the brain, the voiding reflex center, which is at the base of the spinal cord, and the urethral sphincter, the muscle that regulates the flow of urine out of the body. If any of the nerves in this communication system are damaged, various bladder problems can occur, based on where the damage occurs. When the pathways between the brain and voiding reflex center are affected, dribbling, urinary frequency or urgency, or incontinence can occur. This type of damage is common. Two-thirds of MS patients experience some type of bladder problem. Bladder infections also occur often among people who have MS.

Diarrhea and constipation are the two most common bowel problems seen in people with MS. Bowel spasms are the cause of diarrhea, which usually occurs less often than does constipation. Constipation occurs because demyelination in the brain or spinal cord interrupts the nerve messages to the bowel.

VISION PROBLEMS

Problems with vision—blurring, gradual vision loss—are one of the first signs of MS. They rarely affect both eyes at the same time.

COGNITIVE AND EMOTIONAL PROBLEMS

Up to 75 percent of MS patients experience problems with memory and reasoning. Verbal fluency and information-processing difficulties are also common.

BALANCE AND COORDINATION PROBLEMS

Balance and gait disturbances are common and vary in severity. Although the cerebellum is the main center for balance, the spinal cord, eyes, and ears are also involved. The extent of nerve damage in each of these areas determines the extent and seriousness of balance and coordination problems.

SEXUAL DIFFICULTIES

More than 90 percent of men and 70 percent of women with MS report that their sex lives change after onset of the disease. Problems include decreased sex drive, loss of interest in sex, impaired sensation, and reduced orgasmic response.

❖ DIAGNOSIS AND TREATMENT OF MULTIPLE SCLEROSIS: CONVENTIONAL APPROACH

No single test can accurately diagnose multiple sclerosis, therefore doctors need to conduct several tests to help distinguish between multiple sclerosis and other conditions that have similar symptoms (see box, "Oops! Misdiagnosing Multiple Sclerosis," below). Making a diagnosis early in the course of the disease is especially difficult for this reason, and also because nerve abnormalities are not always clear during the early phase. It often takes years for a diagnosis of MS to be reached, and even then doctors often describe the condition as "probable" or "possible" rather than "definite" MS because the disease course is so unpredictable.

Diagnostic Examination and Tests

After the doctor takes your medical history, he or she will conduct a neurological exam. This exam evaluates face and eye movements, reflexes, limb strength, and sensation and coordination. For example, it often includes a test for exaggerated reflexes such as Babinski's reflex, in which the doctor stimulates the sole of the foot and watches for an upward motion of the big toe. An eye examination is conducted for people who have balance and gait problems to determine if there is damage to the optic nerve. At this point, the doctor may use any one or more of the following procedures to help make a diagnosis:

• **Magnetic resonance imaging (MRI).** This is the most sensitive diagnostic imaging technique available; it can reveal areas of the white matter of the brain where lesions have formed as a result of lost or damaged myelin. However, MRI fails to show abnormalities in about 25 percent of people who are in early stages of the disease.

• **Evoked potentials.** This painless test measures electrical responses in the brain when certain nerves are stimulated. For example, you may be shown a flash of light, and your brain's response to it will be recorded via electrodes that have been placed on your head. In people with multiple sclerosis, the response may be slower because the passage of signals along demyelinated nerve fibers is impaired. Evoked potentials shows abnormalities in about 65 percent of cases of early disease.

• **Lumbar puncture.** This test involves using a needle to withdraw a sample of cerebrospinal fluid from the spine. People with multiple sclerosis often have higher levels of white blood cells and slightly higher levels of myelin basic protein and an antibody called immunoglobulin G (IgG) in their fluid. Special lab techniques can be done that separate and chart the various elements in the cerebrospinal fluid to identify a characteristic called oligo-clonal bands, found in about 90 percent of people who have MS.

• **Blood tests.** Although there are no blood tests that indicate multiple sclerosis is present, they may be used to rule out other conditions that mimic MS (see box, "Oops! Misdiagnosing Multiple Sclerosis").

Oops! Misdiagnosing Multiple Sclerosis

Although magnetic resonance imaging (MRI) and other laboratory tests can be helpful in making a diagnosis, doctors still make a misdiagnosis 10 to 15 percent of the time, by either failing to identify MS or misdiagnosing something else as MS.

Diseases with symptoms that are similar to those of multiple sclerosis include:

- Viral or bacterial infections of the brain (Lyme disease, syphilis, AIDS)
- Structural abnormalities of the spine or skull (severe arthritis of the neck, ruptured spinal disk)
- Chronic fatigue and immunodeficiency syndrome (CFIDS)
- Inflammation of the blood vessels in the spinal cord or brain (lupus, arteritis)
- Tumors or cysts of the brain or spinal cord (syringomyelia)
- Lou Gehrig's disease (amyotrophic lateral sclerosis [ALS])
- Small strokes (especially in people who have hypertension or diabetes, who are susceptible to such strokes)

Treatment

Because damage to the nerves can be life-threatening, early treatment is critical. It seems to delay disability, apparently by decreasing the damage to the nerves.

Conventional treatment of MS can be put into three categories: treatment of symptoms, treatment of acute relapses, and use of disease-modifying drugs to treat the underlying immune system abnormality.

TREATING SYMPTOMS

When Carol, a fifty-four-year-old grandmother, opens up her medicine cabinet, it looks like a pharmacy. At various times, she takes more than half a dozen drugs for various symptoms, including bladder problems, pain, spasticity, depression, and tremors. "I reached the point where I was taking drugs to treat the side effects of the other drugs," she says. "And none of them were treating the root of the problem."

Carol's situation is not unusual. There is an arsenal of drugs available to treat symptoms of MS, but all have side effects. For spasticity, for example, the antispasticity drug baclofen is used to calm the nerves in the spinal cord, but it can cause fatigue and weakness. Tizanidine is an option that appears to cause less weakness than baclofen. Another antispasticity drug, dantrolene (Dantrium), is effective but can cause liver damage. Some people resort to injections of botulin, a toxin that causes botulism, the often fatal food poisoning. Injections must be repeated every few months to get relief. Nondrug approaches include stretching exercises, water exercises in a pool, and relaxation techniques.

The chronic pain experienced by some people who have MS is often treated with a class of antidepressants known as tricyclic antidepressants, as well as with anticonvulsants. It is not uncommon for patients to be taking more than one drug for pain. Some of those drugs include gabapentin (Neurontin), lamotrigine (Lamictal), amitriptyline, the anticonvulsant divalproex (Depakote), topiramate (Topamax), and baclofen. Those who experience the extreme pain associated with trigeminal neuralgia are often given phenytoin and carbamazepine, which have a sedative effect. Carbamazepine and phenytoin are also often prescribed for burning, tingling, and crawling sensations, as is the antidepressant amitriptyline.

Tremors are often treated with beta-blockers, antiseizure drugs such as primidone, and tranquilizers, but none of them are very effective. Barbara, a forty-one-year-old accountant, chose to use a brace on her left leg rather than expose herself to the side effects of drugs. The brace reduces the severity of tremor in her right leg so she can walk without fear of falling.

TREATING RELAPSES

Patients in the early stages of MS often get symptoms in the form of attacks or acute relapses, in which a new symptom evolves over time, perhaps weeks or months, and eventually goes away. Each new relapse is a new area of inflammation that has developed, so acute relapses are treated with anti-inflammatory drugs to try to minimize damage. People with milder forms of MS are often given a pituitary hormone known as adrenocorticotropic hormone (ACTH), an anti-inflammatory.

Corticosteroids such as prednisone or methylprednisolone are given for short periods to relieve acute symptoms, and may shorten the duration of attacks. These immunosuppressive drugs have many potential side effects associated with long-term use, such as weight gain, bone density loss, fatigue, and susceptibility to infections. Other immunosuppressive drugs, such as azathioprine, cyclophosphamide, and cyclosporine have not been effective.

DISEASE-MODIFYING THERAPY

Certain drugs are designed to treat the underlying immune abnormality and to reduce the risk of future damage. Drugs in this category that are currently used to treat MS are Avonex, Betaseron, and Copaxone. Avonex and Betaseron are types of a natural immune substance called beta interferon, which may reduce relapses by up to 30 percent among people who are in the relapsing-remitting phase. Common side effects of these drugs include sweating, muscle aches, fever, chills, depression, fatigue, and injection-site irritation, as these drugs must be injected under the skin.

Copaxone is a synthetic form of myelin basic protein, a natural component of myelin, which protects nerve fibers. This drug may reduce the relapse rate by about one-third. Copaxone is injected beneath the skin once a day and can cause injection-site irritation, muscle weakness, tremor, runny nose, and weight gain.

Monoclonal antibodies is an experimental therapy in which the antibodies are targeted at specific cells (T-cells, helper T-cells) that are believed to damage the nervous system in people who have MS. Researchers at Stanford University in California are testing monoclonal antibodies against specific gene types called HLA-DR2, which appear in some people who have multiple sclerosis. This treatment may be available in the near future.

❖ EVALUATION AND TREATMENT OF MULTIPLE SCLEROSIS: MY APPROACH

While conventional doctors are concerned about diagnosing "possible," "probable," or "definite" multiple sclerosis, I focus on identifying the autoimmune process that is underlying and causing the symptoms. After all, when a person is experiencing muscle pain, bowel problems, spasticity, and tremors, they aren't having "probable" or "possible" symptoms; the symptoms are definite, and need to be addressed at their origin.

Evaluating Nadine

Nadine, a forty-year-old wallpaper hanger and painter, had been diagnosed with multiple sclerosis one year prior to seeing me. Her primary complaint was numbness over her entire body. Before coming to the Edelson Center, she had been taking Avonex, but the side effects—fatigue, muscle weakness, fever, and depression—caused her to stop. She had a history of chronic allergies, migraines, mouth ulcers, and chronic conjunctivitis. She also had restless legs syndrome (a condition in which the legs jerk, twitch, and kick uncontrollably at night) and insomnia.

Her environmental history uncovered more than a dozen years of exposure to paints, carpeting, varnishes, fabrics, and other chemically treated materials because of her work. She also had four amalgams and consumed fish several times a week. We conducted several tests to uncover how her immune system was functioning. This is what we found:

- Elevated levels of interleukin-2 and interleukin-4 and gamma interferon, which indicated an overactive immune system.
- Elevated levels on the immune complex study, which is common in MS and other systemic autoimmune conditions (e.g., lupus, CFIDS).
- Elevated levels of anti-Sm antibodies, myelin basic protein, and anti-myelin oligodendrocyte glycoprotein (MOG), all of which are indicative of MS.

- Increase in CD4-CD8 ratio, indicating an overactive immune system.
- Decreased natural killer cell activity, seen in people who have MS as well as other autoimmune disorders.
- High levels of mercury and lead on heavy metal challenge.
- Food sensitivities, including milk and milk products, oranges, peanuts, wheat (gluten, a common allergy among people with MS), and white potatoes. Food allergies are a possible cause and trigger of MS symptoms.

Treating Nadine

Fortunately, Nadine was in the early stages of the disease. As the test results showed, she had many clear indications of MS, plus high heavy metal levels to support the damage being done to her nerve fibers. Her history of chronic allergies could have contributed to the development of myelin nerve damage. I chose the following treatment options for Nadine:

• Chelation therapy. We used DMPS and DMSA to remove the heavy metals from her system. Nadine began her treatment at the Center for one month and then continued it at home for an additional five months.

• Avoidance diet. Nadine eliminated those foods to which she was sensitive and learned to make substitutions, such as soy milk for cow's milk and rye bread instead of wheat. I also recommended that she avoid the following foods, as they can overstress the body: refined sugar; processed, canned, or frozen foods; alcohol; and coffee.

• Environmental controls. I encouraged Nadine to make her home and home office as toxin-free as possible, which included installation of HEPA (high-efficiency particulate arresting) air filters and reverse-osmosis carbon water filters, and the use of natural cleaning products. She removed processed foods from her diet, which eliminated chemical additives, and switched to organic produce. Although her work as an interior designer often placed her in situations with fabrics, paints, and other chemicals, she avoided exposure to these toxins as much as possible.

• Gamma globulin, intravenous. There is evidence that IV gamma globulin promotes remyelination (see chapter 13).

• Nutritional therapy. We added the following supplements: essential fatty acids omega-3 and omega-6 (flaxseed or primrose oil) for their anti-inflammatory effects; sulfur to protect against toxins; vitamin B_{12} (sublingually) to help protect myelin sheaths from damage.

After one year of therapy, Nadine's mercury and lead levels had dropped dramatically and there was a mild improvement in myelin basic protein antibody levels. Both anti-Sm antibody and immune complex results were negative. Her body numbness had disappeared, as had much of the restless legs and insomnia. She was also pleased that her migraines had virtually disappeared, which we attributed to the elimination of the reaction-producing foods from her diet.

❖ WHAT YOU CAN DO NOW

• Find a doctor who performs the tests and uses the treatments discussed in this chapter (see chapter 2).

• Make your home environment as toxin-free as possible (see chapter 11 for specific suggestions). I recommend installation of HEPA filters and water filters, and avoidance of all pesticides, insecticides, herbicides, and household cleaning chemicals.

• Ask your doctor to test you for food allergies and sensitivities. These are possible triggers of MS symptoms.

• Switch to a whole foods, organic diet that includes lots of fruits and vegetables and whole grains. You want to avoid hormones, steroids, and food additives, preservatives, and colorings (see chapter 12).

• Take essential fatty acids in the form of organic, unrefined flaxseed oil, 1 to 2 tablespoons daily.

• Use one or more of the herbal chelators (burdock root, dandelion root, lemon balm, milk thistle, uva ursi, yellow dock; at the discretion of your healthcare provider) listed in chapter 11. Always consult with your healthcare provider before using herbs. I do not recommend use of these herbs as the only biodetoxification approach.

• Consider using the nutritional chelators (glutathione, lipoic acid, cysteine, N-acetylcysteine) listed in chapter 11. Always consult with your physician before taking these supplements, to determine the proper dosage and which ones are most appropriate for you.

• Take antioxidants and other essential nutrients. You can see a list of the suggested supplements and dosages in chapter 12.

❖

Chapter 9

Miscellaneous Autoimmune Disorders

In chapters 3 through 8, we discussed the most common autoimmune disorders, which total less than a dozen. Yet scientists have identified approximately eighty different autoimmune diseases. What about the more than five dozen conditions we haven't included? Although they affect fewer people—and in some cases are very rare—we want to mention at least a few of them because they affect tens of thousands of people in the United States, and because they illustrate further how pervasive autoimmunity is in our population. In fact, people with autoimmune disorders often have more than one autoimmune condition.

In this chapter we share with you information about ten less-common autoimmune conditions. One important message to take with you from this chapter is that there are common threads that run between these and the other autoimmune disorders covered earlier in this book. You will notice that autoimmune disorders have many similar symptoms. This, of course, is one factor that makes it difficult for doctors to diagnose them. But it also is evidence that autoimmune disorders share common causes.

That leads me to the next point. Because *I believe that heavy metal and/or chemical toxicity is a causative factor in nearly every, if not all, autoimmune disorders,* I have not repeated this information under "Causes" in every entry. I do, however, include information about other contributing causes and triggers.

You will also notice that I have not included treatment information in this chapter, except for what is included in the two patient stories. Why? Because *my basic treatment approach for all autoimmune cases* (the disorders in this chapter as well as those in the previous chapters) *is the same: elimination of heavy metals and/or chemicals, with the appropriate nutritional therapy to support it.* Naturally, other treatments are then added, tailored to the person's specific needs. My success with this approach supports the idea that all autoimmune disorders have their origins in an autoimmune process that is triggered by heavy metal and/or chemical toxicity.

❖ ANKYLOSING SPONDYLITIS

Although rheumatoid arthritis is the most common of the rheumatoid disorders, ankylosing spondylitis may be the other condition in this category with which people are most familiar. Ankylosing spondylitis, or arthritis of the spine, is a systemic disease that, unlike most autoimmune disorders, is more common in men than in women. Symptoms appear most frequently in males ages sixteen to thirty-five years. About 300,000 Americans (less than 1 percent of the population) have this condition, and it is three times more common in whites than in blacks.

Signs and Symptoms

Although some people experience symptoms of ankylosing spondylitis in many parts of the body, the lower back is the defining site in this disorder. The onset of lower back pain and stiffness is usually gradual, taking weeks or months. Other signs and symptoms may include loss of appetite, fatigue, fever, joint pain, and damage to the heart, lungs, and eyes. The eye is the most common organ affected by ankylosing spondylitis: 25 percent of people who have ankylosing spondylitis experience eye inflammation (iritis).

Causes

A gene known as HLA-B27, which is found in 8 percent of healthy white Americans and in 2 to 3 percent of healthy blacks, has been identified as making people more susceptible to getting spondylitis. Experts believe that no more than 2 percent of people born with this gene will eventually get the disease, and that other genetic factors play a role in causing other symptoms of spondylitis, such as eye inflammation. If a family member has spondylitis and you test positive for HLA-B27, your chance of getting the disease increases to 20 percent if you are younger than forty, but your risk is much lower if you are older.

Several studies suggest that spondylitis is caused by an infection. In particular, klebsiella, through a process of molecular mimicry (when part of a molecule of one protein resembles part of another totally different protein), are seen in the colon of a high percentage of people who have ankylosing spondylitis. Also supporting the infection link is the fact that people who have this disease are more likely to have genital infections caused by the organisms mycoplasma, chlamydia, and ureaplasma. It's also been noted that nearly everyone who has spondylitis has intestinal changes like those seen in people who have Crohn's disease or ulcerative colitis (see chapter 7).

❖ AUTOIMMUNE HEPATITIS

In 1950, scientists described the first documented case of autoimmune hepatitis, or autoimmune chronic hepatitis, as a disease of young women. What distinguishes autoimmune hepatitis from other types of chronic hepatitis is the presence of autoantibodies, such as those for anti–smooth muscle and antinuclear antibodies (ANAs).

At first, scientists thought the disease was related to lupus (systemic lupus erythematosus) because the two conditions share similar symptoms, including the presence of antinuclear antibodies (ANAs) in hepatitis patients. Later, however, they decided it was a different disease and named it autoimmune hepatitis. Other signs of autoimmune hepatitis include elevated levels of gamma globulin, progressive inflammation of the liver, and chronic hepatitis seen on liver biopsy.

Autoimmune chronic hepatitis most often develops in young women (70 percent of those affected) during adolescence to early adulthood. Women are eight times more likely to get the disease than are men.

Causes

Some people who have the gene types HLA-B8 and HLA-DR3 seem to have a predisposition to develop autoimmune hepatitis. Some research suggests that a virus triggers onset of the disease, but this has not been proven.

Crystal's Story

At first, overwhelming fatigue and aching joints led Crystal to believe she might have chronic fatigue and immune deficiency syndrome or lupus. (In fact, lupus frequently appears with auto-immune hepatitis; see chapter 4.) But when the skin of this twenty-five-year-old social worker began to take on a tinge of yellow, she went to a doctor, who discovered that she had jaundice, as well as an enlarged liver. These symptoms, along with itching, skin lesions (called spider angiomas), and abdominal discomfort, are the classic symptoms of autoimmune chronic hepatitis.

Crystal's doctor did a liver biopsy to confirm his suspicions, as well as an ANA test, which was positive, as it is in 60 percent of cases of autoimmune chronic hepatitis. She also had raised levels of gamma globulin, which is found in more than 80 percent of people with the disease. Crystal's doctor announced that they had caught the disease fairly early and that her prognosis was good. Later stages of the disease are characterized by abdominal fluid and mental confusion, which Crystal thankfully had not experienced.

Conventional Treatment

Crystal had started conventional treatment before she came to my Center. She had been taking the immunosuppressive drug prednisone, along with azathioprine. This combination allows lower doses of prednisone to be used, as prednisone is associated with serious side effects, including hypertension, cataracts, diabetes, and bone loss, as well as weight gain. This drug program is designed to reduce symptoms, improve liver test results, and prolong survival. In up to 75 percent of patients, liver tests do improve to normal range, and Crystal was no exception. However, within three months of stopping treatment, she had a relapse, as the majority of patients do within six months of ending therapy. Because she did not want to go through the drug program again, she came to my Center.

MY APPROACH

My evaluation of Crystal revealed that she had raised levels of mercury and lead, nutritional deficiencies, and oxidative stress. We initiated chelation (DMPS and DMSA) for the heavy metals and several approaches for possible viral infections, including daily supplementation with glycyrrhyzin, a licorice derivative that destroys viruses; ozone autohemotherapy; and thymus extract injections. Crystal also started intravenous mega–vitamin C therapy.

After six months, Crystal's mercury and lead levels were within safe ranges, her liver test results were normal, and she was feeling energetic and healthy. She has been following a healthy (organic) diet and a special nutritional supplement program we developed for her, has instituted environmental controls such as use of water filters in her home and HEPA air filters (see chapter 11), and has not experienced a relapse.

❖ DIABETES (TYPE 1)

Insulin-dependent diabetes mellitus (IDDM) is an autoimmune disease in which the endocrine system—specifically the beta cells in the pancreas—is the focus of attack. For reasons that are not entirely clear (see "Causes," below) the immune system turns against the insulin-producing beta cells (islet cells) in the pancreas and destroys them. (Usually, about 80 to 90 percent of the beta cells are destroyed before a person has noticeable symptoms of diabetes.) Without insulin, glucose (sugar) cannot enter the cells, where it is necessary for energy production in the mitochondria.

Once the body can no longer produce insulin, individuals need to take daily doses of prescription insulin, usually by injection.

About 800,000 people in the United States have IDDM, which represents only about 5 to 7 percent of all cases of diabetes in the country. (The most prevalent form of diabetes—about 90 percent of cases—is noninsulin-dependent diabetes. It typically first appears after age forty, and is not an autoimmune condition.) Scientists have identified several autoantibodies typically seen in people who have IDDM, including those against insulin (these autoantibodies are usually the first ones to appear), islet cells, and a substance called glutamic acid decarboxylase.

IDDM is often referred to as childhood diabetes because it usually first appears during the first twenty years of life. It is more common in females than in males. The incidence of IDDM is higher among individuals who have specific autoimmune diseases, including Hashimoto's thyroiditis, Graves' disease, and pernicious anemia.

Signs and Symptoms

IDDM can be insidious, as the process of beta cell destruction can go on for months or years before symptoms become apparent. Parents need to be aware of the warning signs of IDDM and to bring their child to a doctor as soon as possible should they occur. Symptoms can include frequent urination, fatigue, hunger (even though the child has consumed sufficient amounts of food), unusual thirst, and weakness. Some children have trouble functioning in school and may be restless, irritable, or apathetic, or experience vision problems such as blurred sight.

Causes

Research indicates that most, if not all, people with IDDM may inherit factors that make them susceptible to the disease. However, not everyone who has these inherited traits develops IDDM, thus other factors trigger the autoimmune process. Some scientists believe that that factor may be a virus. Others suggest that leaky gut syndrome triggers the disease process when proteins, such as casein in cow's milk, pass through the gastrointestinal barrier. Antibodies to the casein are believed to react with the beta cell proteins and destroy them.

❖ KIDNEY DISEASE (AUTOIMMUNE)

The kidneys are responsible for filtering the blood, removing toxins and impurities, and producing urine for elimination. Anyone who has chronic renal (kidney) failure can accumulate deadly poisons and die unless they receive treatment. Glomerulonephritis is a form of autoimmune kidney disease that can lead to chronic renal failure. The name refers to structures called the glomeruli, part of the capillary network where filtration takes place in the kidney, and nephritis, inflammation of the kidney. The disease affects about 4 in 100,000 people in the United States. The presence of autoantibodies against an essential part of the filtration process, the glomerular basement membrane, characterizes this autoimmune disease.

Signs and Symptoms

Because most cases of glomerulonephritis develop very gradually, it can take years for symptoms to appear. One classic sign of glomerulonephritis is excess protein in the urine (proteinuria).

However, people would not know they had proteinuria unless it was found during a urinalysis. Some people have blood in their urine (hematuria), which at least is a visual signal that something is wrong, and so their doctor could test them for proteinuria as well. Both of these problems occur because damage to the glomeruli causes insufficient filtering of the blood, which results in blood and protein loss in the urine. Other symptoms of glomerulonephritis may include nausea, vomiting, fatigue, headache, and reduced urine output.

Causes

The causes of autoimmune kidney disease are unclear; however, it is known that exposure to gold compounds (which are used to treat people who have a type of progressive rheumatoid arthritis) and drugs containing mercury can cause a similar disorder. This supports heavy metals being a cause of the disease. Microorganisms are also suspect, although the culprits have yet to be named.

❖ MYASTHENIA GRAVIS

Myasthenia gravis is a chronic autoimmune disease that affects the way muscles respond to signals from nerves. The result is extreme muscle weakness, which can occur anywhere in the body, including the eyes. In order for muscles to move normally, they rely on receiving chemical signals from the nerves. These signals cause the nerves to release a chemical called acetylcholine, which leaves the nerve and attaches to special receptors on muscle cells. Once the receptors have been stimulated by the acetylcholine, the muscle can contract.

In people who have myasthenia gravis, the body's immune system attacks the receptors with antibodies, destroying or blocking them. This action prevents some or most of the chemical signals from getting through, so the muscle cannot contract properly and it becomes weak. (Up to 80 percent of a person's receptors can be damaged.) Thus, one of the diagnostic tests for myasthenia gravis is for acetylcholine receptor antibodies.

One form of the disease affects the eyes only, causing them to have a droopy, sleepy appearance. This type of myasthenia gravis often eventually develops into the more general form, however. Overall, myasthenia gravis most often affects women between the ages of twenty and forty. When it first appears in people older than forty, it affects both males and females equally. It frequently occurs in people who have other autoimmune disorders as well.

Signs and Symptoms

The hallmark symptom of this disease is fatigue that worsens as the day progresses. That means that people may feel and be strong when they first get up in the morning, but as they continue to use their muscles, they become increasingly weak. This is referred to as myasthenic fatigue. The muscles that control the eyelids and eye movements are usually affected first, followed by those that control chewing, swallowing, and talking. Eventually the weakness spreads to the arms and legs, and in some people it affects their ability to breathe. Depending on which muscles are affected, symptoms can include blurred or double vision, slurred speech, shortness of breath, drooping eyelids, and weakness in arms, legs, fingers, hands, and neck.

Causes

Although scientists are not certain what triggers the body's attack on itself, the thymus gland (the master gland of the immune system; see chapter 1) appears to have a role in the disorder. Most people with myasthenia gravis have abnormal thymus function. Infants born to mothers who have the disease have an increased risk of having myasthenia gravis at birth, but the infants' symptoms usually disappear within a few weeks.

❖ POLYMYOSITIS

Imagine feeling so weak that combing your hair is a major accomplishment. People who have severe polymyositis ("poly" meaning "many"; "myositis" meaning "inflamed muscles") can reach that stage of the disease. Polymyositis is an autoimmune disorder that usually strikes children between the ages of five and fifteen and adults between the ages of fifty and seventy. Females are twice as likely as males to get the condition. Muscle weakness may build up gradually over weeks or months, or it may appear suddenly. A similar condition, called dermatomyositis, is characterized by a rash.

It is estimated that polymyositis affects 1 in every 100,000 people in the United States. The disease affects blacks more than it does whites. In most of these cases, the disease is not fatal, but it can be debilitating.

Signs and Symptoms

The main symptoms of polymyositis are muscle weakness, especially in the hips and shoulders, and painful swelling in the small joints. Less common and less severe is muscle soreness. Shortness of breath and difficulty speaking or swallowing affect those whose throat, breathing muscles, lungs, or heart are involved. If these muscles are involved, the condition can be fatal.

Causes

Some researchers suggest that a virus triggers the autoimmune response, but there is insufficient evidence to support this. Heredity may be a factor, as frequently there are cases of polymyositis in one person and another autoimmune connective tissue disease in another member of the same family. However, because polymyositis is not a common disease, a family history of the disorder is unusual.

❖ SCLERODERMA

Scleroderma is a chronic autoimmune disease in which the skin, and more often both the skin and connective tissue (systemic scleroderma), are the targets of the body's attacks. The result of the attacks is tight skin that, if it affects organs, can eventually cause them to fail. In systemic scleroderma, the affected tissues can include the esophagus, intestines, lungs, heart, and kidneys. The most common form of scleroderma, called CREST syndrome, is characterized by tight skin that affects only the hands, but does involve the gastrointestinal tract and lungs. Both men and women get systemic scleroderma, but women are affected more often, especially those between the ages of thirty-five and fifty-four.

Signs and Symptoms

Along with skin thickening, more than 95 percent of people with scleroderma also have Raynaud's phenomenon, in which the small blood vessels in the fingers, toes, and sometimes the nose and ears constrict. The constriction results in these body parts turning white, cold, and numb, followed by a rush of blood that rewarms them and causes pain. Other symptoms may include hair loss; swelling of the fingers, hands, forearms, face, feet, and lower legs; vaginal dryness; joint pain and swelling; muscle weakness; thickening of tendons; heartburn; bloating; shortness of breath; chest pain; kidney damage; dry eyes and mouth; and impotence.

Causes

Scientists have identified several autoantibodies that are typically found in people who have scleroderma. These individuals also tend to have abnormal collections of certain T-cells in the skin and other sites in the body. The antibodies or T-cells damage small arteries, which leak fluid and cause swelling. They also release chemicals that lead to an overproduction of collagen (a fibrous protein), which accumulates and causes the skin and organ linings to thicken, harden, and tighten.

Several triggers have been suggested to cause the autoimmune response that results in scleroderma. One is exposure to certain chemicals, specifically epoxy resins, aromatic hydrocarbons, and vinyl chloride. I believe that many other chemical toxins, plus heavy metals, should be added to that list. Another trigger is the presence of leftover fetal cells circulating in the bloodstream even decades after pregnancy.

❖ SILICONE IMMUNE TOXICITY SYNDROME

About thirty years after silicone breast implants first began to be used, hundreds and then thousands of reports of complications were made. What had started out to be a positive, confidence-boosting operation sought by an estimated two million women turned into an autoimmune nightmare for thousands of them.

That's because the silicone breast implants that had been placed into their chests had leaked. In fact, research shows that after twelve years of use, up to 95 percent of breast implants had deformities such as holes or cracks. Once the silicone left the implant, it traveled through the body and deposited itself in various sites, causing free-radical damage and an assortment of symptoms in some women (see box).

Silicone Immune Toxicity Syndrome and Autoimmunity

Although at first researchers tried to link the symptoms experienced by women who had leaking silicone breast implants to other autoimmune disorders, such as rheumatoid arthritis and lupus, for me and many other scientists, the symptoms pointed to a new disorder. That disorder eventually was named silicone immune toxicity syndrome. Dozens of studies support the validity of this autoimmune disorder. For example:

- Among 176 women with breast implants who were examined at the Hospital for Joint Diseases in New York, 77 percent had chronic fatigue, 65 percent had cognitive dysfunction, 56 percent had severe joint pain, 53 percent dry mouth, 50 percent dry eye, and 40 percent hair loss.
- At Louisiana State University Medical Center at New Orleans, 300 women with implants had developed musculoskeletal complaints. The symptoms appeared an average of 6.8 years after implantation.

- High levels of antinuclear antibodies (ANAs) were found in 10 of 11 women with implants who also had autoimmune symptoms.
- In a study of 111 women (with and without implants), those with implants had a statistically significant increase in anti-silicone antibodies, with the highest levels seen in women who had a ruptured breast implant.
- An Australian study showed that 70 women with silicone implants had elevated levels of autoantibodies to collagen, similar to what is found in women who have lupus or rheumatoid arthritis.
- A study of 50 women with implants showed that 89 percent had fatigue, 78 percent had joint pain, and 38 percent had positive ANAs.
- In 56 women with implants and scleroderma (an autoimmune disease), the scleroderma had developed an average of nine years after implantation. Among these women, 83 percent had ANAs and 77 percent had Raynaud's phenomenon.

Signs and Symptoms

Women who have silicone immune toxicity syndrome often have many symptoms that mimic those of other autoimmune disorders, and have other autoimmune disorders as well. The most common signs and symptoms include the following:

- Rheumatoid arthritis (see chapter 6)
- Sjögren's syndrome (see "Sjögren's Syndrome," below)
- Severe fatigue

- Tingling in the hands and feet
- Memory and cognitive difficulties
- Night sweats
- Muscle inflammation
- Hair loss
- Abdominal pain
- Emotional instability
- Joint and tendon pain
- Multiple chemical sensitivities and food and inhalant sensitivities

Causes

Silicone breast implants contain silicone gel, a synthetic material containing 38 percent silicon. Silicon is a nonmetallic element found in the soil, and is the primary component of glass. Silicone (medical grade suitable for implantation) is a compound in which the carbon has been replaced by silicon. Silicone used for breast implants is placed in a semipermeable membrane envelope for implantation.

As silicone gel leaks from the implants, the material is picked up by macrophages (immune system cells), broken down, and circulated throughout the body. The gel breaks down into silicon and silica, which cause dysregulation of the immune system. The body produces antibodies against the silicon and also against the protein complex (the complex that forms when silicon attaches to protein molecules in various organs), resulting in an autoimmune response.

In addition, the silicone gel stimulates production of free radicals, which damage cell walls, DNA, and enzyme systems. This damage can be pervasive, affecting all organs in the body.

Daria: A Case of Silicone Immune Toxicity Syndrome

Daria came to the Edelson Center after fighting a three-year battle with silicone immune toxicity syndrome. By age forty-five, she had had a successful career as a dentist, but her symptoms were now making it extremely difficult for her to continue to practice. She took a sabbatical and came to my Center.

Comprehensive Medical History Evaluation Questionnaire responses revealed that during the 1970s she developed sensitivities to metals used in her dental practice. In 1987 she had silicone breast implants and was happy with the cosmetic results. In 1996 she had silicone injected into her face, and her troubles started. She lost twenty pounds, developed muscle and joint pain, had frequent urination, fatigue, headache, bruising in her extremities, digestive problems, abdominal pain, bone pain, edema, dry skin, rash, chest pain, belching, irritability, and decreased cognition, among other symptoms.

We administered a battery of tests and found, among other things, candida and klebsiella infections; deficiencies of the minerals selenium, magnesium, and manganese; high levels of mercury and lead; chemical toxicity (specifically to the toxins toluene, xylene, and dichloromethane); autoantibodies to myelin basic protein; and an increased T-cell reaction to silicone and silicon.

Treatment included chelation using DMSA and DMPS for removal of mercury and lead; high-temperature sauna treatment for chemical toxicity;

nutritional therapy to support chelation and chemical biodetoxification, as well as address mineral deficiencies; immunotherapy to balance her immune system (thymus therapy and IV gamma globulin); nystatin (an antifungal) along with a yeast-free diet to fight the infections; and DMSO for inflammation. Within six months, she was 85 percent improved overall. She returned to work full-time and her health continued to improve.

❖ SJÖGREN'S SYNDROME

Depending on the source, an estimated one to four million Americans have Sjögren's syndrome. Either way, the number is significant. Yet if you ask a hundred people if they know what this disease is, chances are only a handful will be able to answer correctly. Sjögren's syndrome is a chronic inflammatory autoimmune disorder in which the immune system produces autoantibodies that attack the salivary, tear, and other moisture-producing glands, destroying their ability to produce moisture.

Although Sjögren's syndrome can affect men and women of any age, 90 percent of cases are in women, usually of middle age or older. Sjögren's syndrome often accompanies other autoimmune disorders, especially rheumatoid arthritis (in 30 to 50 percent of cases), lupus (up to 30 percent), and scleroderma (4 to 5 percent), and it is often confused with these disorders as well. That's because they share many of the same symptoms (see chapter 4 on lupus, chapter 6 on rheumatoid arthritis, and this chapter for scleroderma).

Signs and Symptoms

The most obvious results of the attack on the moisture-producing glands are dry eyes and dry mouth. However, the lack of moisture in joints and throughout other tissues in the body can lead to many more serious conditions, such as chronic infections, arthritis, severe tooth decay, ulcers, heartburn, chest pain, and skin infections. About 25 percent of people with Sjögren's syndrome experience symptoms that affect their kidneys, thyroid, blood vessels, and muscles. In the majority of cases, however, the damage is done to tear ducts, salivary glands, and the vagina.

Causes

Genetics are believed to play a role in Sjögren's syndrome, because it is found more commonly in families that have other autoimmune disorders. Some researchers have suggested that viruses or hormones contribute to the syndrome, but these possibilities have not been proven.

❖ VASCULITIS

Vasculitis is acute or chronic inflammation of the blood vessels, which can occur alone as an autoimmune disorder, as a complication of other autoimmune diseases, or along with an allergic reaction. The condition may be isolated to one site or be systemic, affecting various organs and parts of the body, including the kidneys, heart, and brain. Chronic inflammation of a blood vessel can cause it to narrow inside, obstructing the flow of blood to tissues (known as ischemia), which can lead to damage of tissues (necrosis), the formation of blood clots (thrombosis), or a weakening or ballooning of a blood vessel wall (aneurysm).

Vasculitis comes in many forms, depending on which blood vessels are affected (see "Signs and Symptoms," below), and each form affects a different population. Men are about three times more likely to get polyarteritis nodosa, for example, while Kawasaki disease is seen most often in children. Men and women are equally affected by Wegener's granulomatosis, in which symptoms usually first appear around age forty, while women are more likely to get giant cell arteritis than are men.

Signs and Symptoms

The signs and symptoms of vasculitis vary, depending on the form of the disease a person has. Here's a brief breakdown of a few forms of vasculitis.

• Polyarteritis nodosa. Affects the smaller blood vessels throughout the body. Symptoms include fever, weight loss, weakness, fatigue, headache, abdominal pain, muscle aches, blood in the urine.

• Hypersensitivity vasculitis. Smaller arteries, veins, and capillaries, especially those in the skin, are affected. This form may be triggered by an allergy or it can be part of an autoimmune disorder. Symptoms include joint pain and purple spots on the skin.

• Wegener's granulomatosis. Smaller arteries and veins in the respiratory tract and kidneys are most affected by this form of the disease. Symptoms include malaise, weakness, joint pain, poor appetite, weight loss, rash, symptoms of kidney failure.

• Giant cell arteritis. The larger arteries leading to the head are affected in giant cell arteritis. Symptoms include fever, anemia, headache, malaise, fatigue, poor appetite, joint pain.

• Kawasaki disease. Causes swollen glands in the neck; swelling in the skin; redness of the lips, palms, and mouth; symptoms of heart disease.

Causes

The mechanism behind autoimmune vasculitis is unknown, but research suggests that abnormal immune chemicals accumulate inside the walls of affected blood vessels, which trigger the body to attack these vessels. This autoimmune response produces inflammation and vessel damage. Some cases of vasculitis may be caused by allergy or hypersensitivity to certain drugs, such as penicillin or sulfa, or to inhaled environmental irritants.

❖ WHAT YOU CAN DO NOW

• Find a doctor who is knowledgeable about autoimmume disease and environmental toxins (see chapter 2).

• Make your home environment as toxin-free as possible (see chapter 11 for specific suggestions). I recommend installation of HEPA filters and water filters, and avoidance of all pesticides, insecticides, herbicides, and household cleaning chemicals.

• Switch to a whole foods, organic diet that includes lots of fruits and vegetables and whole grains. You want to avoid hormones, steroids, and food additives, preservatives, and colorings (see chapter 12).

• Ask your doctor to test you for food allergies. Food allergies and sensitivities are common among people who have an autoimmune condition.

• Use one or more of the herbal chelators (burdock root, dandelion root, lemon balm, milk thistle, uva ursi, yellow dock; at the discretion of your healthcare provider) listed in chapter 11. Always consult with your healthcare provider before using herbs. I do not recommend use of these herbs as the only biodetoxification approach.

• Consider using the nutritional chelators (glutathione, lipoic acid, cysteine, N-acetylcysteine) listed in chapter 11. Always consult with your physician before taking these supplements to determine the proper dosage and which ones are most appropriate for you.

• Take antioxidants and other essential nutrients. You can see a list of the suggested supplements and dosages in chapter 12.

Chapter 10

Chronic Fatigue and Immune Dysfunction Syndrome: A "Partial" Autoimmune Disease

In 1984, in the upscale, idyllic resort town of Incline Village, Nevada, on the shores of Lake Tahoe, about two hundred people fell ill with a mysterious disease. The main symptoms were severe fatigue and muscle aches, and the victims were primarily white, wealthy, female, and young. The media latched on to the story, and the strange disease was dubbed "yuppie flu" and "yuppie plague," among other names. Most of the general public, including doctors, didn't take the disease seriously, especially since the symptoms were largely subjective.

But today, the estimated 800,000 to more than one million Americans who have chronic fatigue syndrome, the name given to the disease in 1988 by the Centers for Disease Control and Prevention (CDC), take it very seriously. That's because it can attack any part of the body, at any time, with varying levels of severity, and be debilitating for days, weeks, months, or years. We now know that it definitely does not affect just the wealthy: it crosses all economic, social, ethnic, and age barriers. In an effort to capture the seriousness of this illness, it is now often referred to as chronic fatigue and immune dysfunction syndrome (CFIDS).

Although the term CFIDS is relatively new to Americans, the disease process itself is no stranger to people in many other parts of the world, including Canada, Britain, Europe, Australia, and New Zealand, where there has been a similar syndrome called myalgic encephalomyelitis reported since at least the 1950s. Even before then, a condition referred to as "undue fatigue," or neurasthenia, was described for the first time in the medical literature in 1869.

❖ CFIDS: A TRUE ENVIRONMENTAL DISEASE

Doesn't it seem unusual that there were no reports of neurasthenia before 1869 and that it first appeared when the industrial revolution was just getting under way and introducing pollutants to the environment? Coincidence? We think not. A link between the appearance of CFIDS and the introduction of and then dramatic increase in the number and amount of toxins to which people are exposed has been researched by many scientists and environmental physicians. This idea is just one that supports an environmental cause of CFIDS (see "Causes, Triggers, and Risk Factors," below). Although CFIDS is not the only medical condition that has been linked with environmental toxins—indeed, nearly every one has been—it appears to be one of the ones that was "born" in the toxic age.

❖ CHRONIC FATIGUE AND IMMUNE DYSFUNCTION SYNDROME TODAY

If you have or suspect you have CFIDS, it's hard to tell you how much company you're in. Attempts to determine how many people in the United States have CFIDS have proved difficult. One major problem is that many symptoms are involved (see below), and they can be associated with other medical conditions (for example, lupus, multiple sclerosis, fibromyalgia). Thus doctors must go through a process of elimination and conduct good detective work to get a diagnosis (see "Diagnosis and Treatment of CFIDS: Conventional Approach," below). Other reasons for the air of mystery around CFIDS include a general lack of research on the syndrome and an unwillingness by some physicians to acknowledge that it exists.

According to the CDC, 4 to 10 per 100,000 adults (about 10,440 to 26,100 Americans) have CFIDS, but a 1999 study published in the *Archives of Internal Medicine* found the number to be 422 per 100,000 in general, with a high number (726 per 100,000) among Latinos. Jesse Stoff, M.D., coauthor of *Chronic Fatigue Syndrome: The Hidden Epidemic,* estimates that more than four million people in North America have the syndrome.

The truth is, we don't know how many people have CFIDS. We do know that:

- More women than men have the syndrome, at a ratio of about three to one.
- It affects people of many different racial and ethnic groups, with more Latinos and blacks affected than whites or Asians.
- Symptoms typically first appear in people between the ages of twenty-five and forty-five.

❖ IS CFIDS AN AUTOIMMUNE DISEASE?

Some debate surrounds the question concerning whether CFIDS is an autoimmune condition. I, for one, believe that *while CFIDS has characteristics of autoimmunity, it is not a true autoimmune disease.* We discuss it in this book because it has autoimmune characteristics.

The American Autoimmune Related Diseases Association says that the presence of antinuclear autoantibodies (ANAs) in many people with CFIDS suggests, but does not prove, that it is an autoimmune process. (You will learn, in fact, that high levels of ANAs are common among many people who have different autoimmune disorders.) Another bit of evidence that supports the autoimmune idea is the discovery of autoantibodies to a component of human cells called lamin B-1.

According to the National Institute of Allergy and Infectious Diseases, CFIDS appears to involve interactions between the immune and the central nervous systems, and admits that these are interactions scientists do not understand well. Yet many professionals seem to agree that CFIDS occurs in people who have a genetic predisposition for autoimmunity.

❖ IS CFIDS CONTAGIOUS?

If viruses are involved in CFIDS, they probably can be transmitted to other people. Clusters of CFIDS cases, like the one at Incline Village in 1984, suggest that the syndrome could be contagious. However, the vast majority of people who are in close contact with people who have CFIDS do not develop the syndrome. The deciding factor is believed to be whether an individual is susceptible to autoimmunity and to whatever triggers are responsible for causing the disease in that particular person (see "Causes, Triggers, and Risk Factors," below).

❖ CAUSES, TRIGGERS, AND RISK FACTORS

Chronic fatigue and immune deficiency syndrome is a complicated, multifaceted disease that is likely caused by several factors working together. If we accept the idea that CFIDS involves autoimmunity, something must trigger the disease process, and one of the most debated theories has been that a virus is responsible.

A Viral Connection?

In the past, the Epstein-Barr virus, a herpes-like virus believed to cause infectious mononucleosis, was suspected, for several reasons: it can cause many of the same symptoms seen in people with CFIDS, and some people with CFIDS have high levels of Epstein-Barr antibodies in their system. However, Epstein-Barr virus has largely been eliminated as a candidate because many people with CFIDS do not have the antibodies, and the virus is relatively common among the general population, the vast majority of whom do not have CFIDS.

I believe that a large number of people with CFIDS may have Epstein-Barr virus *secondary* to depression of part of the immune system that leads to reactivation of infection that was previously present in the cell. Using PCR technology (see "Infectious Organism Evaluation," in chapter 2), it is possible to locate the DNA of this and other organisms that are suspected to be part of CFIDS.

Some researchers propose that substances called mycoplasmas, the herpesvirus-6, or *Chlamydia pneumoniae* set off the process. Mycoplasmas have been linked with Gulf War illnesses, and the latter two organisms have been associated with multiple sclerosis, all conditions that have symptoms similar to those seen in CFIDS. Other scientists suggest that enteroviruses or retroviruses are involved. The role of all these organisms in CFIDS has yet to be determined. However, I believe that all these mycoplasmas and viruses, including Epstein-Barr, are merely part of CFIDS and not the cause.

Environmental Factors

I, along with many of my colleagues, believe that environmental factors such as heavy metals and chemicals can be at the root of this disease process, and our beliefs can be verified using lab studies (see "Evaluation and Treatment of the CFIDS Autoimmune Process: My Approach," on p. 223). Toxins such as mercury, lead, formaldehyde, aluminum, and pesticides cause immune system dysregulation and excessive oxidative stress, or directly damage the cells themselves, which eventually brings about chronic fatigue and other symptoms of CFIDS, depending on which organ systems are damaged.

Stress Factor

Physical trauma and even severe emotional stress have been suggested as triggers for CFIDS. However, the Centers for Disease Control and Prevention, along with the Chronic Fatigue and Immune Dysfunction Syndrome Association of America, announced in March 2001 in a consensus panel that stress probably did not cause CFIDS. "But," said panel chair Dimitris A. Papanicolaou, M.D., of Emory University in Atlanta, "there's a lot of evidence that stress can exacerbate [CFIDS] if it's already there." I believe that CFIDS is exacerbated by the increase in cortisol levels (a stress hormone that at high levels, can cause fatigue) as well as the rise in free-radical production.

The CFIDS Autoimmune Process

The CFIDS autoimmune process probably begins with a genetic predisposition that is related to a problem with detoxication—likely with damage to a system of cellular enzymes called the 2'5'a-synthetase system. This damage could be initiated by chemical toxins, heavy metals, and/or infections. Once the damage begins, it leads to an increase in substances called alpha interferons, which are known to cause autoimmunity. Other effects follow, including a decrease in the efficiency of messenger RNA, which causes a decline in the ability to fight infection, and a decline in cellular metabolism. The result is that every cell in the body can become involved in the autoimmune process, affecting various systems and causing problems such as:

- Visual disturbances
- Muscle weakness and fatigue
- Abnormal functioning of the liver, which means the body's ability to rid itself of toxins (detoxication process) is hindered
- Heart failure and arrhythmia
- Hearing loss
- Seizures and ataxia

The answer to what causes CFIDS may be any or all of the possibilities discussed here, in any given individual. Although we don't have any definitive answers yet, the bottom line is that cells are damaged by environmental toxins (e.g., pesticides, heavy metals, various toxic chemicals, infectious organisms, drugs, alcohol),

causing organs to malfunction and illness to develop in susceptible individuals.

❖ SIGNS AND SYMPTOMS

The hallmark of CFIDS is overwhelming, persistent, incapaci-
tating fatigue that leaves those affected unable to carry on their
normal physical functions. The source of this fatigue is mitochondrial dysfunction—the result of damage from chemicals,
heavy metals, and other toxins to the mitochondria, which are the
energy sources of cells. This fatigue is not relieved by rest or sleep,
cannot be explained after clinical evaluation, and is a new development rather than something that has been a lifelong complaint. After this primary criterion is met, the Centers for Disease
Control and Prevention (CDC) requires that four or more of the
following symptoms be present in order for a diagnosis of CFIDS
to be made. The CDC states that these symptoms must have per-
sisted or recurred for six months or more and must not have appeared before the fatigue.

- Short-term memory problems
- Concentration difficulties
- Sore throat
- Swollen or tender lymph nodes
- Muscle ache and pain
- Pain in multiple joints without redness or swelling
- Recurring headaches that are different in severity or pattern
  from those experienced previously
- Sleep that does not leave you feeling refreshed
- Post-exercise malaise that lasts more than twenty-four hours

But what if you have debilitating fatigue, along with only two of the other symptoms, but other specific complaints, such as visual problems, constipation, chronic yeast infections, indigestion, depression, or any of the other many symptoms often associated with CFIDS (see box, below)? Does that mean you don't have CFIDS?

If you want an "official" diagnosis of CFIDS, then no, you don't. But for me, the bottom line is this: it doesn't matter if someone has "enough" symptoms to be diagnosed with CFIDS or if we assign a label to every person who has symptoms of CFIDS. If an autoimmune process is occurring—and autoimmunity is just one aspect of CFIDS—and people's lives are being affected, we need to identify the problem and help those individuals. I believe that the root of CFIDS is contamination with toxic heavy metals and chemicals, and that is the villain that must be addressed.

Other Symptoms Associated with CFIDS

People with CFIDS often also have other symptoms, including:

- Visual disturbances (blurred vision, sensitivity to light, eye pain)
- Psychological problems (depression, anxiety, panic attacks, mood swings, irritability)
- Chills and night sweats
- Shortness of breath
- Balance problems, dizziness, lightheadedness
- Bowel problems (diarrhea, constipation, intestinal gas, abdominal pain)

- Numbness, tingling, and/or burning sensations
- Low-grade fever
- Sensitivity to heat and/or cold
- Irregular heartbeat
- Rashes
- Menstrual problems (PMS, endometriosis)
- Dry mouth and eyes
- Ringing in the ears (tinnitus)
- Sensitivity to odors, sound, chemicals, and medications
- Muscle twitching
- Seizures
- Fainting

❖ COURSE OF THE DISEASE

The course of CFIDS and the extent of disability can be as varied as the people who develop the syndrome. For many people the course is like a roller-coaster, with periods of feeling better followed by times when symptoms worsen or new ones appear. How long each of these up and down times lasts differs from person to person and even for the same individual. For some people, the down times grow progressively longer and the symptoms progressively worse.

There are no reliable figures on how many people recover from CFIDS, and one reason for this lack of data is that there is uncertainty about how "recovery" is defined for this condition. Does it mean that people return to the full level of functioning they had before getting the disease, without any relapses, or does it mean near full functioning with periodic relapses? According to a CDC study in which researchers are monitoring people who have had CFIDS for more than five years, approximately 50 percent of patients report they recovered, with patients defining "recovery" for themselves.

❖ DIAGNOSIS AND TREATMENT OF CFIDS: CONVENTIONAL APPROACH

The majority of people who are experiencing the symptoms of CFIDS seek help from conventional doctors who, if they believe CFIDS exists, make their diagnoses based on the criteria set by the CDC, and then treat symptoms. This is the approach most patients can expect and the one with which they are familiar. The results, however, will be less than satisfying, because conventional medicine fails to address the root of the problem, and thus the CFIDS never goes away. It lives up to its name—chronic.

In this section we discuss how conventional doctors diagnose and treat CFIDS and look at the strengths and weaknesses of their approach. Then, in the next section we explore my approach to evaluation and treatment, which delves into the core of the problem—the autoimmune process—and how this comprehensive method can bring lasting relief to people with CFIDS.

Diagnosing CFIDS

"Getting a diagnosis was nearly as much of a nightmare as having the disease is," says Jeannette, a forty-one-year-old former elementary school teacher. When she went to her doctor complaining of chronic fatigue, muscle aches, and headaches, her doctor told her there was nothing wrong and to "take naps." "How could I take naps?" she asked. "I was teaching all day!" She sought help from two other doctors before she located one who believed she had a "real" medical problem. Soon, Jeannette found herself undergoing endless tests.

TYPICAL TESTS

The tests Jeannette refers to often include those in the accompanying box. They are conducted because there is no one diagnostic test or indicator that can clearly identify CFIDS. Another difficulty in diagnosing CFIDS is that symptoms tend to fluctuate, rising and falling in severity, sometimes disappearing for a while, only to return later (see "Course of the Disease"). These drawbacks, along with the fact that symptoms of CFIDS are similar to those of many other disorders (e.g., lupus, hypothyroidism, Lyme disease, fibromyalgia), means that doctors must test for and then rule out other conditions. Sometimes people discover that they have CFIDS and another disorder as well.

"I discovered that getting a diagnosis was a process of elimination. I felt like I was guilty until proven innocent: I was 'accused' of having dozens of other diseases, and as test results eliminated them, we narrowed the diagnosis down to CFIDS," says Jeannette.

Typical Conventional Tests to Diagnose CFIDS

Here are some of the most common tests conventional doctors perform when testing for CFIDS. (The actual tests your doctor uses may differ.) These tests provide useful information, and I usually use most of them as part of my evaluation process. However, they provide only the tip of the iceberg, whereas my evaluation digs to the core of the problem (see "Evaluation and Treatment of the CFIDS Autoimmune Process: My Approach").

• **Complete blood count (CBC).** Helps rule out leukemia, anemia, and other blood disorders as well as collagen vascular disorders such as lupus.

• **Blood chemistry.** Confirms normal blood sugar, renal and liver function, electrolytes, calcium and bone metabolism, and serum proteins.

• **Thyroid function.** Confirms normal thyroid function, a common cause of muscle aches and fatigue.

• **Sedimentation rate.** Indicates the presence of inflammation, infection, and collagen vascular disorders.

• **Urinalysis.** Excludes infection, renal disease, and possibly collagen vascular disorders, such as lupus.

• **Antinuclear antibody (ANA).** This test is typically used in the diagnosis of lupus and other autoimmune processes. Because lupus and CFIDS share many of the same symptoms, the ANA is often given to rule it out.

• **Lyme serology.** Measures the presence of Lyme disease antibodies. Lyme disease and CFIDS share many of the same symptoms. However, this test is usually only given to people who may have been exposed to this tick-carrying disease, which is largely in the eastern part of the United States.

• **Tilt table testing.** Done to identify the cause of dizziness and fainting. Up to 96 percent of people who have CFIDS occasionally experience a sudden decline in blood pressure when standing from a reclining position (orthostatic hypotension) or a rapid rise in heart rate with the same activity (orthostatic tachycardia). It is a relatively expensive test, however, and so is not always done. The reason this study is positive in nearly all patients with chronic fatigue is that toxins have damaged their autonomic nervous system, which is responsible for blood pressure regulation, among other functions.

Conditions That Share Some Symptoms with CFIDS

The following conditions share many symptoms with CFIDS. Note that most of them are autoimmune disorders (not all of them are discussed in this book, as some of them are rather rare), which supports the similar-symptoms, similar-cause, similar-treatment approach I use.

Addison's disease	Hyperthyroidism
Anemia	Hypothyroidism
Anxiety disorder	Irritable bowel syndrome
Behçet's syndrome	Lupus
Celiac disease	Lyme disease
Crohn's disease	Multiple sclerosis
Cushing's syndrome	Muscular dystrophy
Diabetes	Myasthenia gravis
Exposure to toxic chemicals,	Polyarteritis
pesticides, heavy metals	Reiter's syndrome
Fibromyalgia	Rheumatoid arthritis
Giardiasis (parasitic infection)	Sjögren's syndrome
Hepatitis	Ulcerative colitis

Treatment

Once a diagnosis of CFIDS is made, the majority of doctors announce to their patients that it's time for treatment, which in most cases means drugs designed to mask symptoms. Unfortunately, none of them will relieve all the symptoms or eliminate the underlying cause of this disease.

DRUGS

Medications can be given to provide symptom relief: the more symptoms you have, the more drugs your doctor may prescribe. A characteristic of people with CFIDS is that they are unusually sensitive to drugs, which often means they must take doses that are much lower than the standard ones. Another consideration is that while some drugs may be very helpful to some patients, they are little or no help to others. Even those drugs that provide relief for a while may abruptly stop being effective.

Thus, you may find yourself with a medicine cabinet full of prescription and over-the-counter drugs for pain and flulike symptoms (e.g., ibuprofen, naproxen, acetaminophen), depression and fatigue (e.g., fluoxetine [Prozac], sertraline [Zoloft], paroxetine [Paxil]), indigestion (lansoprazole [Prevacid], ranitidine [Zantac]), sleep problems (tricyclic antidepressants such as doxepin and amitriptyline), and other complaints.

LIFESTYLE CHANGES

Conventional doctors often recommend lifestyle changes in addition to drugs and other medical treatments for CFIDS. These steps, which can be taken by anyone who has CFIDS, can improve the quality of life.

"This disease has changed my entire life," says Tanya, a twenty-nine-year-old former dancer. Not only has CFIDS caused her to quit the career she loved, but she has had to find support from among a whole new set of friends. "My dance friends sympathize, but they have active lives," she says. "I can't keep up with them anymore." She sees a therapist twice a month to help her battle the depression and attends support group meetings when she has the energy to do so.

The emotional stress and depression associated with CFIDS are a critical part of the vicious cycle of the disease: people are depressed because they have debilitating symptoms, and depression fuels fatigue. Some people with CFIDS find that stress management (e.g., relaxation exercises, yoga, meditation), cognitive behavioral therapy, and sleep management therapy help them deal with the emotional aspects of the disease.

Modifications to lifestyle are rarely an option: people with CFIDS usually find that their symptoms force them to reduce or eliminate many of their activities. However, there are positive changes you can make that will help you better manage and live with CFIDS. They include:

- If you smoke, stop.
- If you drink alcohol, stop.
- Improve your diet, eat whole natural foods, organic when possible, and eliminate junk food, fatty foods, and sugars.
- Develop some type of nonaerobic exercise program. (Aerobic exercise can be counterproductive, because it increases free-radical production and damages the mitochondria.) Yes, we know you have fatigue, but moderate exercise helps raise serotonin levels, which in turn reduces fatigue. Ten minutes of stretching several times a week and a slow (about 2 miles per hour) fifteen-minute walk three to four times a week can actually make you feel energized. Naturally, if you are in the midst of a severe period of fatigue, the fifteen-minute walk should be bypassed until you feel better.
- Get eight to ten hours of sleep per night, go to bed before 10 P.M., and get up at the same time every morning. Schedule a thirty-minute nap during the day.

• Manage your stress. Meditation, yoga, and tai chi are good stress busters. Spend at least fifteen minutes a day managing stress.

❖ EVALUATION AND TREATMENT OF THE CFIDS AUTOIMMUNE PROCESS: MY APPROACH

Unlike the tests conducted using a conventional medicine approach, which are done to arrive at a diagnosis, the evaluation procedures I use are performed to determine the underlying causes for diagnoses like oxidative stress, nutritional deficiencies, allergic/sensitivity reactions, gastrointestinal dysfunction, and hormonal dysfunction, so that the proper treatments can be started to return the individual to a healthy state.

To understand CFIDS, it is necessary to take a "holistic," total-body approach. That means we need to study the biochemistry of the affected individual and his or her environment, including invading organisms, nutritional deficiencies, enzyme deficiencies, allergies, hormone levels, digestion, exposure to heavy metals and chemicals, and stress, to see what is happening at a cellular level. All of these factors can cause oxidative stress, which can damage the cells in various parts of the body.

To uncover what is happening at the molecular level in patients who come to me with symptoms of CFIDS, I choose from dozens of test options. I make my selections based on what I uncover during the extensive general evaluation process. Because it is not practical to list and explain all of the tests I may administer to individuals who have CFIDS symptoms, those listed below are a representative sample. This list gives you an appreciation of the many directions a thorough investigator must go to understand the autoimmune process in CFIDS. Each of these tests is explained in chapter 2.

- Heavy metal challenge
- Chemical toxicity evaluation
- Infectious organism evaluation (viral studies using PCR for mycoplasma, candida, chlamydia)
- Intestinal permeability evaluation
- Gastrointestinal evaluation (CDSA and lactulose mannitol challenge)
- Oxidative stress panel
- Nutritional studies (vitamin, mineral, organic acid, and amino acid levels)
- Sensitivity evaluation (blood and skin testing for allergies/sensitivities)
- Immune system evaluation and immune system activation of coagulation test (for hypercoagulable characteristics—increased coagulation of the blood)
- Nervous system evaluations, if indicated

Roberta

When Roberta came to me, she was so ill she had to lie on the couch during the entire ninety minutes it took for me to gather her history. At age thirty-nine, Roberta had a lifelong history of headaches and allergies. In her mid-teens she had developed irritable bowel syndrome, and three years before coming to see me the chronic fatigue had started. Along with overwhelming exhaustion came muscle weakness, muscle spasms, and difficulty with memory. Other symptoms soon followed, including (but not limited to) eczema, hearing loss, tinnitus, dry mouth, swollen lymph glands, abdominal bloating, nausea, diarrhea, lack of coordination, dizziness, depression, and irritability.

Although there was nothing extraordinary about Roberta's childhood environment, about four years before her first visit to my office she and her husband had realized a dream: they had bought a new home on a golf course, where they could engage in their favorite pastime. Unfortunately, their dream appeared to be a nightmare for Roberta, because both the house and the golf course were exposing her to a constant barrage of pesticides, herbicides, solvents, and other chemical toxins.

Roberta had visited several doctors who claimed to be specialists in chronic fatigue, but none of them had helped her or had ever done comprehensive testing. Because of her extensive list of symptoms (more than thirty-five) and her history, she was a candidate for many of the diagnostic tests available.

When I compiled the results, they showed a picture of a very active autoimmune process. She met the criteria for CFIDS and had severe nutritional deficiencies; multiple chemical sensitivity; leaky gut syndrome; allergies to food, preservatives, and other substances; chemical toxicity; mercury toxicity; autoimmune encephalopathy (mental confusion); autoimmune thyroid binding autoantibody production; and several other diagnoses. Roberta would be a treatment challenge, but not one that couldn't be met.

Treating CFIDS: My Approach

Multifaceted disease processes like CFIDS must be dealt with on an individual patient basis. Each patient who comes to me is treated using a program that is developed based on the findings of the evaluation. Thus, if two forty-year-old women, both with a prior diagnosis of CFIDS, come to me for treatment, I evaluate what is happening at a cellular level for each woman and then select treatments based on those findings.

Generally, my therapeutic approach includes techniques to accomplish the following:

- Remove any of the toxins that were discovered during the evaluation
- Provide the body with the nutrition it needs to allow the cells to work efficiently again
- Initiate remedies that will heal damaged organs

Some of the techniques are things you can do for yourself; others require the assistance of healthcare professionals. The individual treatment programs presented here are examples only; not only is each person's autoimmune process unique, but his or her entire biochemical makeup and biological functioning as well. Therefore your treatment program would be tailored to your specific needs. You can see how my approach works by looking first at how I treated Roberta, whom you met above, and then at another case, Charlotte.

ROBERTA

One of the first things Roberta needed to do was to remove herself from her toxic environment: out of her new home and away from the chemical-ridden golf course. Unfortunately, she and her husband did not want to give up their dream, so we tailored her treatment around her circumstances.

Here is an overview of Roberta's treatment program. Details on individual therapies are in part III.

• Environmental controls. Even though Roberta refused to leave her toxic environment, we took measures to minimize the toxic stress. She installed HEPA (high-efficiency particulate arresting) filters in her home (capable of removing nearly 100 percent of all pollens, molds, spores, dust, and particulates from the air) and water purifiers on her faucets. I also recommended that she use only natural cleaning supplies in their home (e.g., baking soda, vinegar, lemon, borax) and place air-purifying plants (e.g., English ivy, bamboo palm, mums) indoors to absorb toxins from the air.

• Ultraviolet blood irradiation. This therapy improves immune function and inactivates viruses that are in the bloodstream.

• Growth hormone therapy. This was initiated to help boost energy level, enhance the healing process, improve immune function, and improve memory.

• Chelation using DMPS and DMSA. Both DMPS and DMSA are substances that are used to remove toxic heavy metals from the body.

• Food avoidance diet. We developed an eating plan that eliminated the foods and food additives to which Roberta was intolerant or allergic.

• Progesterone therapy. Roberta's hormonal tests revealed low progesterone levels, which contributed to her fatigue, depression (progesterone is a natural antidepressant), irritability, bloating, and dizziness.

• Nutritional therapy. Roberta needed both oral and intravenous nutritional therapy to restore her natural detoxication system (the liver). She was started on a regimen of antioxidants, mineral therapy, amino acid therapy, and various other supplements, including but not limited to calcium d-glucurate, acetyl L-carnitine, amrit kalash, beta-glucan, ginkgo biloba, essential fatty acids, phosphatidylcholine and serine, glutathione, N-acetylcysteine, lipoic acid, naringinine, thymus extracts, SAM-e, methyl-cobalamine, and other substances. As you can see, a great many nutrients are needed to correct this complex autoimmune process. (See glossary for definitions.)

• High-temperature sauna therapy. Roberta's chronic exposure to chemicals made this therapy critical. She underwent routine sauna sessions to help rid her body of chemical toxins.

• Gastrointestinal healing therapy. A program of probiotics (supplements of healthy bacteria), glutamine, aloe vera, and antifungal and antibacterial factors were needed to address Roberta's leaky gut syndrome, which was depleting her body of essential nutrients as well as causing diarrhea and gastrointestinal distress.

It took nearly eighteen months of continuous therapy, but Roberta was feeling 90 percent better by that time. Because Roberta apparently has a predisposition for autoimmunity, it would be best for her to avoid toxic environments as much as possible.

CHARLOTTE

Charlotte was a forty-year-old overweight mother of a ten-year-old boy. She had a history of about twenty years of various health problems, some of which included chronic fatigue, eczema, chronic sore throat, wheezing, night sweats, abdominal cramping, diarrhea, muscle pain, leg cramps, sensitivity to chemicals and certain foods, and headache. Her symptoms had started during her sophomore year in college, and by the beginning of her senior year the fatigue, muscle aches, and headaches were so bad she had to drop out.

After I evaluated Charlotte and got back her test results, they showed that she had type II diabetes, elevated blood levels of the pesticide DDE and mercury, signs of oxidative stress, a yeast infection, deficiencies of magnesium, calcium, potassium, selenium, and phosphorus, and hypersensitivity to many foods, trees, grasses, dust and salicylates (aspirin and similar drugs).

I drew up a treatment program for Charlotte, and after discussing it with her, she started on the following (each treatment approach is discussed more fully in part III):

• Avoidance diet. Charlotte was sensitive to wheat, corn, peanuts, and milk and dairy products. We removed them from her diet and found substitutes (e.g., rice and rye products for wheat; soy milk and soy cheese for dairy).

• Environmental controls. She installed water and air filters in her home and converted to organic produce and grains.

• Immunotherapy. Charlotte underwent eighteen months of EPD vaccine treatment to eliminate her many allergies.

• Chelation. She was put on a program of chelation with DMPS, a substance that helps remove various metals from the body.

• Nutritional therapy. Charlotte was seriously deficient in several minerals, so in addition to adding a mineral supplement to her program, we also included antioxidant therapy to tackle the oxidative stress and promote liver function to better detoxify her body. We added niacin, chromium, and vanadium to stimulate the processing of carbohydrates and fats, which would help with her weight problem and diabetes.

• Anticandida therapy. Both a yeast-free diet and an anti-candida program, including grapefruit seed extract, were added to eliminate the systemic yeast infection.

Charlotte felt better within just a few months of beginning treatment. After eighteen months, she reported feeling 90 percent better than when she had first come to me. She has reenrolled in college to finish the degree she gave up on more than two decades ago.

OTHER TREATMENT OPTIONS

Depending on the needs of the patient, other treatment options I may use include herbal products that modulate the immune system (immunomodulating products), acemannan (an extract from the aloe vera plant), bio-oxidative therapy (ozone, hydrogen peroxide), transfer factor, and thymus extract (see part III). Discuss these options with your physician.

❖ WHAT YOU CAN DO NOW

• Find a doctor who performs the tests and uses the treatments discussed in this chapter (see chapter 2).

• To manage stress, muscle pain, and fatigue, try massage, tai chi, and acupuncture, which have been used successfully by some patients.

• Make your home environment as toxin-free as possible (see chapter 11 for specific suggestions). I recommend installation of HEPA filters and water filters, and avoidance of all pesticides, insecticides, herbicides, and household cleaning chemicals.

• Switch to a whole foods, organic diet that includes lots of fruits and vegetables and whole grains. You want to avoid hormones, steroids, and food additives, preservatives, and colorings (see chapter 12).

• Ask your doctor to test you for food allergies.

• Use one or more of the herbal chelators (burdock root, dandelion root, lemon balm, milk thistle, uva ursi, yellow dock; at the discretion of your healthcare provider) listed in chapter 11. Always consult with your healthcare provider before using herbs. I do not recommend use of these herbs as the only biodetoxification approach.

• Consider using the nutritional chelators (glutathione, lipoic acid, cysteine, N-acetylcysteine) listed in chapter 11. Always consult with your physician before taking these supplements to determine the proper dosage and which ones are most appropriate for you.

• Take antioxidants and other essential nutrients. You can see a list of the suggested supplements and dosages in chapter 12.

Part III

TREATING AUTOIMMUNE DISEASES

Biodetoxification:
How to "Clean Your House"

This chapter addresses one of the three cornerstones of my treatment approach to autoimmunity. It's about cleaning house—literally and figuratively. We're going to talk about flushing toxins out of your body, vacuuming your living space, filtering your water, and cleaning up your air and food supply. We're cleaning out environmental toxins, because they create free radicals, and free radicals are at the core of autoimmunity. Heavy metals and chemicals—such as pesticides, formaldehyde, benzene, and others found in household cleaners, cigarette smoke, food additives, and hundreds of other products—are not welcome visitors in our bodies or our homes. When they invade the body, they create free radicals, cause physical and emotional symptoms from headache to depression, and, in susceptible individuals, can cause auto-immunity.

The more scientific term for this housecleaning is biodetoxification. Biodetoxification is any process that removes toxins—

heavy metals and chemicals—from the human body. This removal is especially critical for people who have an autoimmune condition, because the toxins fuel their autoimmunity process.

In this chapter I'll explain the biodetoxification program we use at the Edelson Center as well as a program you can use at home, after consulting with your doctor. These methods are, in my opinion, a critical and necessary part of healing from autoimmune disease.

But before we can explain the various ways to remove heavy metals and chemicals from your body, you need to understand the enemy better—just what are these toxins and where do they come from?

❖ HEAVY METALS AND CHEMICALS

Would you want a toxic dump in your neighborhood? How about one in your backyard, your office, or your living room? Chances are, there is a dump in each of those places right now. In the name of progress, we are dumping thousands of tons of toxins into our environment every year. They are in our air, our food, our soil, and our water. They lurk in our clothing and in our furniture, in the walls of our homes and in the paper we write on, and they are leaking out into the air. Our bodies make heroic efforts to deal with these toxins and to eliminate them.

But sometimes the burden is just too much. For different people, that breaking point—the point at which toxins cause significant cell damage and disease—is different. Factors such as heredity, lifestyle, nutritional habits, and overall state of health, especially that of the immune system, help determine how much impact those toxic substances will have on each one of us.

Make no mistake: toxins affect everyone at some level, even though many people do not realize that their fatigue, headache, dizziness, aches and pains, indigestion, and dozens of other symptoms have their roots in environmental toxins. But for tens of millions of people, those environmental substances are triggers for autoimmunity.

Heavy Metals

The heavy metals most often found at unacceptable levels in the body are aluminum, arsenic, cadmium, lead, mercury, nickel, and tin. Once in the body, heavy metals have an affinity for the immune system, where they can cause much free-radical damage.

How are we exposed to these heavy metals? Here's just a partial list:

- Arsenic: tap water, herbicides, insecticides and insecticide residue on fruits and vegetables, wood preservatives, automobile exhaust, paint, and cigarettes
- Aluminum: tap water, antiperspirants, baking powder, stomach antacids, household pots and pans, maraschino cherries, toothpaste, dental amalgams, cigarette filters, tobacco smoke, laxatives
- Cadmium: cigarette smoke, tap water, evaporated milk, paint pigments, silver polish, fertilizers, fungicides, rubber, and rubber carpet backing
- Lead: leaded gasoline fumes, paint, canned food with lead seams, meat and milk from animals that have been fed lead-contaminated food, atmospheric lead from coal burning and automobile exhaust
- Mercury: fish, amalgam fillings, mascara (especially waterproof), contact lens solution, fabric softeners, batteries with mercury cells, fungicides for lawns and plants, calamine lotion, and tap water

- Nickel: hydrogenated vegetable oils, peanut butter, margarine, kelp, oysters, herring, cigarette smoke, tea, batteries
- Tin: coated food cans, processed foods, industrial waste, air pollution

Chemicals

An estimated 60,000 different chemicals are in our environment—in our food, air, water, soil, and everyday objects. According to the Natural Resources Defense Council, for example, 845 million pounds of poisonous chemicals were applied to American crops in 1997. Here are just a few of the toxic chemicals we are exposed to each day and their sources:

• Benzene: found in cigarette smoke, gasoline, inks, oils, paints, plastics, rubber, detergents, explosives, pharmaceuticals, and dyes. One study estimates that 45 percent of our exposure to benzene comes from cigarettes, especially if you smoke or if you are exposed to secondhand smoke.

• Chloroform: found in cleaning solvents, floor polishes, insecticides, artificial silk, and lacquers.

• Dichlorobenzene: found in deodorants, insecticides, metal polishes, mothproofing, lacquers, and paints.

• DDT (dichlorodiphenyl-trichloroethane): this pesticide, which was outlawed in the United States in 1972 because it is extremely toxic, can still be found in soil and other substances, including—according to a study done by the Southwest Research Institute in the 1990s—carpeting. The Institute discovered that 90 of 362 midwestern homes examined by their investigators had DDT in the carpeting, likely brought into the homes on the soles of people's shoes.

• Formaldehyde: found in nearly all indoor environments.

Foam insulation, particle board, pressed wood products, grocery bags, waxed papers, facial tissues, paper towels, wrinkle resisters, adhesive binders in floor coverings, backings on carpet, and cigarette smoke contain formaldehyde.

• Hexane/heptane/pentanes: found in glue, cement, adhesives, paint thinner, plastics, gasoline, ink.

• Toluene: found in petroleum products, carpets, carpet glue, copy paper, paint.

• Trichloroethylene (TCE): your dry-cleaned clothes may be making you ill: more than 90 percent of the TCE produced is used in dry-cleaning products and metal degreasers. TCE is also used in printing inks, lacquers, varnishes, adhesives, and paints. The National Cancer Institute lists TCE as a liver carcinogen.

• Xylene: found in rubber, paint, ink, photo-processing products, plastics, insecticides, petroleum products.

Mercury: A Toxin of Mammoth Proportions?

Charles Williamson, M.D., codirector of the Toxic Studies Institute in Boca Raton, Florida, is very outspoken when it comes to mercury. He believes that in the near future, "mammoth" lawsuits concerning the use of mercury dental fillings (amalgams) will be even bigger than the lawsuits now being filed against the tobacco industry. "Mercury vapor is toxic, period," he says. "Specifically, mercury vapor can cause learning disabilities, autism, and attention deficit disorder in unborn children." He also notes that mercury toxicity can appear as a long list of symptoms, including irritability, restlessness, emotional instability, loss of memory, muscle weakness, loss of coordination, abdominal cramps, chronic diarrhea and/or constipation, abnormal heart rhythms, repeated infections, chronic headache, allergies, joint and muscle pain, unsteady gait, and depression. Do these symptoms sound familiar?

Both Dr. Williamson and his colleague Jordan Davis, M.D., believe that mercury toxicity related to mercury amalgams is a significant factor in the tremendous increase in learning and behavioral problems, autism, and many other conditions, including autoimmune disorders (specifically lupus, arthritis, multiple sclerosis, and Hashimoto's thyroiditis), that have occurred since the 1940s, the period that corresponds to the widespread adoption of amalgams.

The World Health Organization states that no level of mercury can be considered to be safe. (This is not surprising, especially as mercury is the second most toxic element in the universe, next to plutonium.) I, and many other health professionals, agree with that statement. Yet most dentists, and the American Dental Association (ADA), continue to insist that mercury fillings are not dangerous. They say that mercury vapors that can leak out of the fillings do not pose a threat to health. The ADA's Council on Scientific Affairs 1998 report states that "The Council concludes that based on available scientific information, amalgam continues to be a safe and effective restorative material." Yet dozens of studies and thousands of researchers do not agree. The use of mercury amalgams is clearly a controversial topic and one that doctors, dentists, and researchers will continue to debate for some time. See the appendix for a list of organizations and Web sites that can keep you up-to-date on the issue.

> *Note:* You have a choice! There is a nontoxic alternative to amalgam called a composite filling, or "white filling." They are readily available and offered by many dentists. If you need a dental filling, ask your dentist to do a composite. One reason we are so concerned about amalgam fillings today is that they were the only type of filling offered for many decades, thus most people have them. They are also less expensive than composites, which makes them more attractive. All of this means many individuals have mercury in their mouths and that it may be leaking vapors into their bodies.

❖ THE BODY'S NATURAL DETOXICATION PROCESSES: WHAT GOES ON INSIDE?

For biodetoxification to be successful, it is important for the body's natural detoxication processes to work together and to be in optimal condition. (Note: "detoxication" is the scientific term for the natural *detoxification* process that occurs in the body.) The organs involved in the body's processes are the liver, circulatory system, skin, adrenal and thyroid glands, kidneys, and bowel (gut). The entire process is very complex but important for you to understand so you can appreciate how biodetoxification can help you. So here's a brief description of how the body's natural detoxication process works.

The Liver: The Ultimate Housecleaner

The liver performs two critical functions: it processes nutrients, and it processes and eliminates toxins from the body. It does this by filtering the blood: at any one time, about 25 percent of all the blood in the body is circulating through the liver. That equals about two quarts every minute. Ideally, we should allow the liver to work in a balanced environment. That means, we should eat wholesome foods and in moderation; we should keep our gastrointestinal tract eubiotic (in a state of healthy balance of good and bad bacteria) with probiotics (see chapter 12); and we should avoid exposure to toxins as much as possible. In that way, we (hopefully) will not overburden the liver and prevent it from performing optimally.

Unfortunately, most people don't live that way. When we eat too much, the liver works overtime to process the excessive amounts of nutrients. When we eat foods that are overly processed, contain lots of chemicals, or are contaminated, the liver must detoxify these added toxins along with all the heavy metals and chemicals to which we are exposed from other sources, which also damage the organs. The result is that the liver is overworked, and it is unable to properly detoxify the body.

Liver detoxication is a very complex task that is carried out in two stages called phase 1 and phase 2. A brief explanation of these phases is given in chapter 2 under "Detoxification Evaluation." The ability of these two phases to function properly is critical for detoxication and, subsequently, biodetoxification to work, therefore we perform tests to evaluate these phases.

The Circulatory System

The circulatory system includes both the blood and the lymph. When it comes to detoxication, one of the main functions of the blood is to transport nutrients to the liver, which the organ needs to function properly, and to bring toxins to the liver. The lymph also transports nutrients.

The Skin

Toxins can leave the body through the skin when we perspire. This is the reason why high-temperature saunas are used as an integral part of my biodetoxification program.

The Adrenal and Thyroid Glands

The adrenal and thyroid glands must function efficiently because the hormones they secrete ultimately affect metabolism, and an inefficient metabolism hinders the detoxication process.

The Bowel

The bowel is an avenue for the elimination of toxins in stool. But those toxins can only be eliminated properly if the intestinal muscles are toned, there are lots of good bacteria present, and stool is able to move through quickly. Thus, if you have leaky gut syndrome (a condition in which the intestinal lining is damaged, creating a "sieve"-like environment that allows toxins, bad bacteria, and other disease-causing organisms to leak out of the bowel into the bloodstream; see chapter 12) or constipation, for example, the detoxication process will be hampered. If toxin-containing stool doesn't keep moving through the bowel, the toxins can be reabsorbed by the body and reenter the bloodstream or various tissues throughout the body. In people with autoimmunity, this constant reassault with toxins creates more and more free radicals and thus more damage.

The Kidneys

The kidneys filter blood and produce urine, which is 95 percent water, which is then passed out of the body. Everyone needs at least two quarts of water (64 ounces) daily to support the elimination of chemicals through the kidneys.

❖ BIODETOXIFICATION AT THE EDELSON CENTER

At the Edelson Center, our biodetoxification program benefits people who have a heavy metal and/or chemical burden in their bodies. My experience with autoimmunity has been that nearly every person I've treated who is experiencing an autoimmunity process has had toxic levels of one or more of these poisons. Our program promotes the elimination of toxins through the primary organs of detoxication, which are the liver, skin, bowels, and lungs. Patients sometimes feel dizzy, weak, shaky, and nauseous at times during the detoxification process, but these symptoms are temporary and part of the healing process. Anytime poisons are removed from the body (think about the detox process for alcoholics and drug addicts), these temporary reactions can be expected. The reward, however, is good health.

Below are the basic elements of my biodetoxification program. The program we offer is very complex, and we tailor each element according to the specific needs of each patient that comes to our Center. We realize that this program is not within the physical (we are in Atlanta, Georgia) or financial reach (it is costly and quite often not covered by insurance) of most people. However, we believe it is important for you to know about the program because:

• It demonstrates that it is possible to successfully treat autoimmune conditions when you use techniques that reach to the core of the origins of the illness.

• Knowledge can start you on your path to recovery. You can take the information presented in this book and seek out other doctors who offer some or all of these treatment options.

• It shows you that even though you may not have access to our specific program, you can use other methods, which we explain for you, to detoxify your life and improve your immune system health.

The Program at the Edelson Center

Here are the main elements of the four-week biodetoxification program offered at the Center. Details on each of these treatment approaches are provided in the paragraphs following this list.

• Chelation. Individuals who undergo a heavy metal challenge test (see chapter 2) and show that they have toxic levels of mercury, lead, or other heavy metals undergo chelation treatments. Anyone with autoimmunity who has metal toxicity must have the metals removed in order to heal, and chelation is the most effective way to achieve this. We use both oral and intravenous chelation at the Center. Several herbal and nutritional approaches, although less effective, can be used by people who do not wish to undergo medical chelation (see "On Your Own: Biodetoxification You Can Do at Home").

• High-temperature sauna therapy. A high-temperature sauna up to four times a day is used for individuals who have tested positive for chemical toxicity. A high-temperature sauna draws chemical toxins out of the body. Saunas can also be done at home, but (I recommend) under a doctor's supervision.

• Exercise. Patients typically have three to four easy exercise sessions (at least ten minutes each) per day of treatment at the Center.

• Nutrition therapy. A custom-designed nutritional therapy program is created for each patient we see at the Center and is based on the individual's unique biochemical makeup. Both oral and intravenous supplementation is used. Individuals who undertake a biodetoxification program of their own need nutritional therapy as well. Some suggestions are provided in chapter 12; however, I recommend that you consult a knowledgeable professional to help you.

• Massage. A ten-minute fat massage (one that simply massages the fat and not the deep muscles) is enjoyed by each of our patients after each exercise session. Although massage is not a critical part of a successful biodetoxification program, it's the part that patients enjoy the most. Fat massage helps move toxins out of storage in the body and also reduces tension and stress. I recommend that people get a massage whenever possible.

• Colon hydrotherapy. This treatment option is prescribed for a limited number of patients. If you are doing your own biodetoxification and want to pursue colon hydrotherapy, I suggest that you first talk with your doctor and then have a specialist do it for you. I do not recommend using any of the intestinal cleansing products that are available over the counter.

• Ozone therapy. I use ozone therapy in a great number of patients, because one of its many functions is to indirectly help eliminate toxins from the body by improving immune system functioning. However, because it is primarily an immunotherapy technique, it is discussed in length in chapter 13.

Generally, 40 to 50 percent of toxins are removed from the body after twenty sessions (four weeks) of this intensive program. Then, when patients are ready to leave the Center, they receive an individual program to follow at home. Some of the suggestions in those individual programs—plus many others—are things you can do yourself, today, to help rid your body of toxins and to live a more toxin-free life. Read all about them in "On Your Own: Biodetoxification You Can Do at Home."

High-Temperature Sauna Therapy

"It is hot, incredibly hot, but you just feel like the poisons are leaping out of your body. It's so cleansing." That's how Charlotte, a thirty-five-year-old woman with chronic fatigue and immune deficiency syndrome (CFIDS), described the high-temperature sauna treatments she was getting to help eliminate the pesticides from her body. Charlotte's family had been in the dry-cleaning business, and she had worked in the store with her parents, starting at the tender age of eight and continuing until she left for college. Ten years of chemical exposure had left its mark as CFIDS.

During a sauna treatment session at the Edelson Center, you sit in a cedar, chemically nontoxic sauna that is heated to 150°F. This is the temperature that activates the chemicals deep within the tissues in the body where they hide and cause cellular damage. The chemicals then enter the bloodstream or lymphatic system and are carried to the liver, where they are processed and sent out to leave the body through stool, urine, sweat, or saliva.

At the Edelson Center, the first few sauna sessions last ten to fifteen minutes and are gradually increased until each session is thirty minutes, with three to four sessions per day. While a four-week program of sauna treatments is an excellent start to removing chemicals from the body (about 75 percent can be eliminated during that time), patients are sent home with instructions on how to continue treatments at home as part of a larger, long-term detoxification program. These patients have periodic blood tests to monitor the toxic chemical levels and the progress of their therapy.

Chelation Therapy

Chelation therapy is a method of eliminating heavy metals and minerals from the body. It is used extensively throughout Europe and other parts of the world, less so in the United States, though it is also growing in acceptance here. From the Greek word *chele*, which means "claw," chelation therapy involves infusing "claw-like" molecules into the body, which then grab on to the molecules of things like lead, mercury, and tin—dangerous toxic metals that lead to the production of free radicals, which damage the body—and carry them out of the body in urine, stool, or sweat. (Now you see why high-temperature saunas aid chelation.)

CHELATION: NOTHING TO FEAR

When people hear the word "chelation," many think of blood filtering. True, that is one way medical chelation is performed. In fact, people with heart disease who receive chelation (a common use of the therapy), undergo intravenous (IV) treatments that can last several hours each, and they often need upwards of fifty treatments or more.

The good news is that much of the chelation we use for heavy metal removal does not involve IV treatments at all. In fact, if you read "A Look at the Chelators," you will see that the two chelators we use most often—DMPS and DMSA—are given as capsules, via injection, and/or suppository. One chelator, EDTA, is given intravenously, but it is used only in certain patients.

If you can't or don't want to use medical chelation, there are herbal and nutritional chelators you can use at home. Although they are less effective than medical chelators, they can be very helpful when used as part of a biodetoxification program. Read about them and other parts of a personal biodetoxification program in the section "On Your Own: Biodetoxification You Can Do at Home."

CHELATION IN THE UNITED STATES

Many physicians have seen the wisdom of chelation therapy since it was first introduced in the United States in 1948, when it was used as a treatment for workers who experienced lead poisoning in a battery factory. Shortly thereafter, the U.S. Navy used chelation for sailors who were exposed to lead while painting government ships and docks. Chelation has been used in the United States for several decades for people who have coronary artery disease and other circulatory problems. It is also the treatment of choice for children and adults who have lead poisoning. Today, doctors who practice clinical molecular medicine or environmental medicine are using chelation to remove heavy metals from their patients.

CHELATION IS NATURAL

The chelation used by doctors to rid the body of heavy metals is similar to the chelation process that occurs in our bodies naturally all the time. For example, hemoglobin, the red pigment in the blood that carries oxygen, is bonded, or chelated, to iron. Vitamins, minerals, and trace elements are chelated to other substances as they move throughout the body. There are also many chelators that occur naturally in the body, including lipoic acid, glutathione, N-acetylcysteine, and cysteine (see "Nutritional Chelators," below).

Thus medical chelation performed by doctors is not a foreign or unnatural process. The difference with the artificial method is that we use man-made chemicals (e.g., DMPS, DMSA; see below) whose purpose is to bond with the toxins and escort them out of the body. When used along with lifestyle and dietary changes, including nutritional supplements, chelation can elimi-nate virtually all heavy metals from the body.

Chelation also offers other advantages, which are clearly ben-eficial for people with autoimmunity. Among those benefits are: it lowers high blood pressure, reduces free-radical activity, im-proves memory, relieves extremity pain, and improves blood flow to the organs.

A Look at the Chelators

Once chelators are in the bloodstream, they bind with the metals and leave the body in urine, stool, or sweat. A series of treatments is needed in order to remove all the heavy metals. The majority of people undergo chelation therapy without any difficulties. However, people who have mild or moderate kidney problems should be mon-itored closely during treatment to avoid overloading the kidneys. Anyone who has a severe kidney problem should not receive EDTA.

DMPS (2,3-dimercaptopropane-1-sulfonate) was first developed in China and then was introduced to the former Soviet Union, Japan, and Germany, where it has been used since the mid-1970s. It is now also used in the United States for removal of mercury, lead, arsenic, cad-mium, nickel, tin, and other metals. DMPS can be taken orally, intravenously, or in a suppository. Typically, treat-ment begins with once-weekly injections (some begin with a suppository) for as long as it takes to help clear the bulk of heavy metals from the body. Patients usually receive a heavy metal challenge test every four months to check levels. If the levels have been reduced to a safer range, then oral or suppository chelation therapy can replace the IV treatments until the levels are near zero.

Because DMPS also binds with essential minerals, including copper, zinc, and manganese, it is usually necessary to receive supplements (typically orally; occasionally IV) to replace the minerals that are lost during treatment. Side effects to DMPS are rare and temporary when they do occur and include dizziness and general weakness, caused by a lowering of blood pressure. More common are flulike symptoms, which can appear after the first treatment. These symptoms can last for several days, but can be significantly improved by taking 1000 to 2000 mg vitamin C daily for several days. Currently, DMPS is available in the United States only through a compounding pharmacist.

DMSA (2,3-dimercaptosuccinic acid) is usually given to remove mercury, lead, and arsenic from the body. One feature that makes DMSA different from DMPS is its ability to cross the blood-brain barrier, which means it can chelate with heavy metals that have reached the brain; DMPS cannot. This ability, I have found, makes it especially useful when treating children who have autism (see chapter 3).

DMSA comes in capsules. Treatment courses vary from patient to patient, and can involve either oral or rectal dosing. Most people tolerate DMSA well, but mild side effects do occur, including diarrhea, nausea, vomiting, appetite loss, and rash. A rare side effect is neutropenia (an abnormally low number of neutrophils, a type of white blood cell that helps fight bacterial infections). Because DMSA also chelates the essential nutrients copper, manganese, zinc, and molybdenum, supplements of these minerals are necessary during treatment. DMSA can also indirectly cause deficiencies of magnesium, cysteine (an amino acid), and glutathione (an important antioxidant), so these may need to be supplemented as well.

EDTA (ethylene diamine tetraacetic acid) is given intravenously through a small vein in the arm. It is used to remove metals such as aluminum, cadmium, lead, and tin, but is not effective for removal of mercury or arsenic. Therefore, EDTA is used only in a select number of patients.

Intravenous chelation is painless and in most cases, causes very little discomfort. An intravenous session can last from ninety minutes to three hours and is done while you sit or lie back in a reclining chair. The number of sessions needed to eliminate toxins from the body varies, depending on the patient. Typically, twenty to thirty treatments are needed. Side effects may include dizziness, headache, mild nausea, or irritation at the IV site.

Exercise

You always hear about all the benefits of exercise, and now you can add one more to the list: it helps move chemicals out of your body more easily. However, people who have chronic diseases, such as autoimmune conditions, do *worse* if they engage in aerobic exercise, because it increases production of free radicals. Therefore, our patients do about ten minutes of *easy* aerobic exercise, such as using the treadmill, bicycling, or running in place, before each sauna treatment. Once patients return home, I recommend that they continue with the ten-minute easy exercise only, just before their sauna.

Massage

After the sauna treatment, patients take a shower to wash away the toxins brought to the surface of the skin. This is followed by a fat massage, which usually lasts fifteen minutes. Again, I encourage patients, once they leave the Center, to continue getting a massage as often as possible, as it helps to move chemicals out of fatty tissue into the bloodstream and lymph.

Colon Hydrotherapy

Colon hydrotherapy is recommended for some patients. It is not uncommon for undigested food and waste to harden in the large intestine, where it can remain for weeks, months, or years, putrify, and produce toxic substances. Colon hydrotherapy removes these toxic substances from the colon by gently infusing warm water into the colon via a flexible tube inserted into the rectum. Patients lie on a comfortable treatment table during the entire process, which takes about forty-five minutes. The procedure is done by a professional colon hydrotherapist. The therapist may also massage the abdominal area to help dislodge toxic material in the colon.

Typically, three separate sessions are needed to achieve maximum cleansing. Unlike an enema, which cleans the rectum only, colon hydrotherapy cleans the entire large intestine. To accomplish this, about 25 to 35 gallons of water are transported into and out of the colon during each session. Colon hydrotherapy also improves the passage of nutrients into the bloodstream, provides a favorable environment for good bacteria in the intestinal tract, and helps restore normal bowel movements.

Because colon hydrotherapy stirs up toxins, some people experience minor nausea or fatigue after the session. Any discomfort usually disappears within twenty-four hours. Drinking peppermint tea or applying a warm heating pad to the abdomen can help.

❖ ON YOUR OWN: BIODETOXIFICATION YOU CAN DO AT HOME

Naturally, not everyone who has an autoimmune condition or who wishes to do biodetoxification can come to the Edelson Center. (I do, however, extend the invitation!) If you have been diagnosed with or suspect you have an autoimmune disease, you can take this book to a knowledgeable physician, who can help you with a treatment program that includes biodetoxification. If you want to "clean house" using biodetoxification methods you can do at home, we offer some guidelines in the pages that follow.

As a general precaution, it is always best to consult with your physician before starting any new treatment program, herb, or supplement. I also suggest that you try as many of the methods that appeal to you, and incorporate as many of the environmental controls ("Environmental Controls: Cleaning Up Your Life") as you can.

Herbal Chelators

For centuries, herbalists have known about the detoxification abilities of various herbs, and modern research has shown them to be effective. Although use of these herbs is not as effective as a medical biodetoxification program, they do help eliminate toxins from your body, regardless of which autoimmune condition you may have. Use one or more of them daily (discuss this with your healthcare provider), either as a supplement (a capsule, tincture, or extract; follow package directions) or as an infusion or decoction (a strong tea; directions provided). A slightly different approach is to do a coffee enema (see box, below). Always consult with your healthcare provider before using herbs. I do not recommend use of these herbs as sole therapies for biodetoxification. All can be found in most health food stores.

• Burdock root (*Arctium lappa*). This herb helps cleanse the blood and liver and promotes the elimination of toxins through the kidneys. To make a decoction, boil 24 ounces of water and add 1 tsp root. Cover and steep for 30 minutes. Drink one to two cups daily at room temperature.

• Dandelion root (*Taraxacum officinale*). This lawn nuisance stimulates the elimination of toxins from all cells in the body. To make an infusion, add ½ tsp dried leaves to one cup boiling water and let it steep for 15 minutes. Drink up to three cups per day.

• Lemon balm (*Melissa officinalis*). This herb helps cleanse the lymphatic system. To make an infusion, pour 8 ounces boiling water over 1 to 3 tsp lemon balm leaves. Cover and steep for 10 minutes. Drink two to three cups daily.

• Milk thistle (*Silybum marianum*). This herb protects the liver against the damaging effects of chemicals, medications, and free radicals. Capsules are recommended over other forms: 150 mg three times daily.

• Uva ursi (*Arctostaphylos uva-ursi*). This herb cleanses the lymphatic system. Prepare an infusion by boiling 2 cups water and letting it cool slightly. Then pour the water over 1 ounce dried herb and let it steep for 15 minutes. Drink up to three cups daily at room temperature. If you use the tincture, take 10 to 40 drops in water up to three times daily.

• Yellow dock (*Rumex crispus*). Yellow dock cleanses the blood, liver, and lymphatic system. To make an infusion, pour 16 ounces boiling water over 2 tsp dried herb. Cover and steep for 10 minutes and drink up to three cups daily. If you choose the tincture, take 3 to 4 ml in water three times daily.

Coffee Enema

Coffee enemas have been used for more than a century as part of a general detoxification approach. The strength of coffee enemas is that they stimulate the liver and gallbladder to release toxins and wastes, which enhances the liver detoxication function.

Coffee enemas are safe to do every day; however, you should discuss this treatment with your doctor before you begin, and consult with him or her throughout the course. To prepare a coffee enema, use 2 tablespoons of coffee per quart, organically grown if possible (see appendix). The cleanest commercial brand is Folgers Regular and is an acceptable second choice.

The water should be purified with a reverse-osmosis carbon filtration system; store-bought spring water is an acceptable substitute. Prepare the coffee in a stainless steel or glass coffeemaker (not aluminum, which is toxic). The prepared coffee will be used at body temperature, so you can make it the night before. You may need to heat it slightly if it is too cool.

To prepare for the enema, purchase an enema kit

---

from a drugstore or pharmacy. Fill the enema bag with the body-temperature coffee. Lubricate the colon tube with KY jelly or a similar substance. Lie on your left side and insert the tube slowly about 12 to 18 inches into your rectum. If it kinks, pull it out and try again. Release the stopper on the bag and allow about 16 ounces of coffee to slowly flow in, then reclamp the stopper. Hold the coffee about ten minutes before expelling it. You may find this difficult to do at first, but you will improve with practice. Repeat the enema, holding the coffee for another ten minutes.

It is not unusual to feel slightly jittery after the first few enemas. However, if this feeling continues after the third enema, reduce the strength of the coffee next time.

Nutritional Chelators

The following supplements are mild chelators and can be used at home as part of a biodetoxification program. Exact dosages should be determined by your physician. See chapter 12 for more information about how some of these nutrients, which can be found at most health food stores and pharmacies, are used as part of a nutritional therapy plan.

• Glutathione. This antioxidant protects against free-radical damage by detoxifying substances such as heavy metals and chemicals into less toxic forms. See chapter 12 for more on this important antioxidant.

• Lipoic acid. This sulfur-containing vitaminlike antioxidant is produced by the body. However, there can be a deficiency, depending on environmental conditions (e.g., the presence of toxins) and age. It has proved effective in aiding the detoxication process and in eliminating heavy metals.

• Cysteine. This amino acid is a chelator and a precursor to glutathione.

• N-acetylcysteine. This antioxidant is a precursor to glutathione and is produced from the amino acid cysteine and procysteine. It is a natural sulfur-containing substance with the ability to detoxify various drugs and poisons, as well as mercury, lead, and cadmium.

Nutritional Therapy

Because nutritional therapy is such a big and complex part of biodetoxification, we have dedicated an entire chapter to it (chapter 12). Nutritional therapy includes more than taking vitamins and minerals; it also involves knowing how to choose healthy foods and which foods to avoid; and which other supplements, such as enzymes, probiotics (good bacteria), amino acids, and other substances are important for proper biodetoxification and for healing from autoimmune disorders.

High-Temperature Sauna Therapy

If possible, I recommend that people who are serious about biodetoxification get a home sauna. A home sauna (health club saunas usually are not hot enough, nor are they nontoxic) can provide health benefits for everyone in the family, not just the individual with autoimmunity. For it to be beneficial, however, you need to get a sauna that is made without glues or other toxins (see appendix). Home sauna treatments should not exceed thirty minutes per day and should always be carried out under medical supervision.

Massage

Naturally, a daily or weekly massage is not feasible or affordable for many people, but even once a month is helpful. A massage is an excellent way to release tension and stress, which facilitates the healing process. While you are getting a massage, it is an excellent time to practice meditation or relaxation techniques, such as visualization.

If you do continue with massage, make sure you are getting a fat massage, not a deep, penetrating massage that works the muscles. That type of massage can be harmful to people who are harboring toxins.

Exercise

Before you decide to skip this section, I want to tell you that I'm *not* going to tell you to start a regular aerobic exercise program. On the contrary: aerobic exercise is potentially harmful to people who are playing host to heavy metals and chemical toxins. While you are doing a biodetoxification program at home, you should limit yourself to ten to fifteen minutes of *easy* exercise, such as slow walking (at a 2- to 3-mile-per-hour pace) or stretching. Once you are feeling better—you have significantly less fatigue and your test results show that your chemical toxin and heavy metal levels are within a safe range—then you can begin an aerobic program. Only your doctor can tell you when you're ready for that step.

Colon Hydrotherapy: Alternatives

Although the approaches discussed in this section are supposed to be "things you can do at home," I cannot with good conscience recommend that anyone use any of the over-the-counter home colonic kits or intestinal cleansing programs on the market. Use of these products can prove dangerous, especially if you have ulcerative colitis, Crohn's disease, appendicitis, or hepatitis. If you and your doctor have agreed that colon hydrotherapy should be part of your biodetoxification program, you should go to a professional colon hydrotherapist for your own safety and peace of mind. Your doctor or the hydrotherapist can then make sure you also get the supportive nutrients and probiotics you need to balance the bacterial flora in your intestinal tract.

Environmental Controls: Cleaning Up Your Life

Although there's nothing you can do to change your genes if you are predisposed to autoimmunity, you can significantly reduce the chances that your immune system will attack your own cells. The goal is to be as chemical- and toxin-free as possible—a tall order in today's world, when you consider that we are surrounded by chemicals.

Even if you follow a biodetoxification program that includes all the elements we discuss in this chapter, you still need to make sound choices in your food and water and be aware of your environment, every day, long after you've completed a biodetoxification program. Minimizing exposure to metals and chemicals is important for everyone, whether you have an active autoimmune problem or not, to achieve optimal health. To help you do that, here are some ways to clean up your life.

CLEANING HOUSE

We like to think of our homes as havens, safe places to live and play and raise our children. Yet the pollution level inside most homes is many times higher than that of the air outside, even in polluted areas.

If you find that hard to believe, just look at all the sources of toxins in a home. Carpets, furniture, plastics, foam rubber, upholstery, tiles, linoleum, paint, and varnishes are sources of chemicals such as formaldehyde, toluene, xylene, hexanes, benzene, and others, all of which evaporate into the air that we breathe. Then consider other sources, including household cleaning products and detergents, insecticides and pesticides sprayed in and around the house, and the additives in the food we eat, and it becomes clear that we need to clean house.

How do we do that? Here are a few suggestions:

• Remove toxic cleaning supplies, such as synthetic soaps, detergents, perfumed products, cleaning chemicals, and polishes. Use natural ingredients instead, which not only cost less but are friendly to your health and that of the planet, such as borax, vinegar, lemon, and baking soda. Read *Staying Well in a Toxic World,* by Lynn Lawson; also see my book *Living with Environmental Illness* and other sources (see appendix) for information and suggestions on natural cleaning.

• Use only nontoxic paints, varnishes, and stains in your home.

• Use natural soaps, shampoos, and deodorants.

• Avoid synthetic materials or chemically treated materials for clothing and bedding, which include dry-cleaning. Do not use fabric softeners or detergents that contain formaldehyde.

• Read food labels for undesirable ingredients (see "Read Labels," below).

• Don't smoke, and don't allow others to smoke in your home. Cigarette smoke, first- and secondhand, generates free radicals.

• Vacuum often, and use a vacuum with a dust sensor, which can sense when no more particles can be extracted from the carpet. Carpeting, especially plush and shag carpeting, is a prime reservoir for all kinds of toxins that can be brought into the house on human and pet feet. Removing your shoes when you walk into the house is one way to cut down on the level of toxins in carpeting. Wiping your feet on a commercial-grade doormat can also reduce the amount of toxins brought into the house.

READ LABELS

Have you ever seen the commercial in which a young boy is trying to read the ingredient list on a container of ice cream, and he is stumbling over the long chemical names? Then another little boy picks up a different ice-cream container and reads off ingredients like milk, cream, and chocolate? When was the last time you read the ingredient list on the foods you eat? The product labels on many foods on supermarket shelves today read like chemical experiments. And they are recipes for disaster to your body. You may think that a little artificial food coloring, preservative, or flavoring won't hurt, but when you consider that you probably eat many foods with these ingredients every day, year after year, that adds up to a big assault on your immune system. One solution is to eat whole, natural foods whenever possible, organic when you can get it.

Don't stop with food labels. Read labels on household products such as shampoos, mouthwash, antiperspirants, detergents, toothpaste, and lotions. Many of these products contain metals such as mercury, lead, and aluminum, as well as other chemicals.

CLEAN WATER, CLEAN AIR

Chances are, the water running out of your tap contains elements you don't want in your drinking water. Mercury, lead, arsenic, fluoride, chlorine, and dozens of other chemicals and microorganisms may be invisible to the eye, but not to your body. I typically recommend that my patients install water filters in their home. The most affordable water filter that will remove microorganisms as well as synthetic chemicals and heavy metals is a reverse-osmosis carbon block filter.

Many people buy bottled water, believing that it is superior to tap water. However, toxins from the plastic bottles can leach into the water, especially if the bottles have been left in the heat. Also, much bottled water is not regulated, and so you can't be sure that synthetic chemicals have been removed.

You may not have a lot of control over air pollution outside, but you can control your inside air quality. I recommend that patients install HEPA (high-efficiency particulate arresting) filters in their homes, or at least in their bedrooms. There are portable units you can take to your office as well. Other suggestions include:

• Put pollution-reducing plants in living and work spaces. These include bamboo palm, mums, English ivy, Chinese evergreen, corn plant, diffenbachia, spider plant, and wandering jew. These plants remove chemicals such as formaldehyde, benzene, and trichloroethylene from the air.

• Have your heating and air-conditioning system cleaned and inspected regularly and replace filters every few months.

• If possible, replace carpets with tile or wood.

• Avoid cigarette smoke (don't allow people to smoke in your home); stores that sell fabric, carpet, furniture, or building supplies; and newly painted or carpeted rooms.

• Use only nontoxic methods of pest control, such as boric acid or thermal heat treatments, the latter of which must be done by professionals.

• Avoid using oven cleaners, drain cleaners, and toilet bowl cleaners that contain chemicals. Use natural methods only (see appendix).

RUN FROM RADIATION

Most of us don't think about the many different ways we are exposed to radiation every day of our lives. High-level radiation, largely in the form of X-rays we get from our dentists and doctors, is the most recognizable source. The unnatural frequencies caused by these radiation sources can damage molecules in the body and stimulate the formation of free radicals. Yet many people believe that even low- and mid-level radiation, such as that emitted by appliances, power lines, cellular phones, computers, and other electric sources can also cause free-radical formation. This is a controversial topic, and scientists on both sides of the issue are convinced they are right.

I believe that low- and medium-level radiation, and definitely high-level radiation, have an effect on cell functioning and free-radical formation. Certainly the cumulative effect of being exposed to multiple sources of radiation may aggravate autoimmunity. Therefore, I encourage my patients to avoid exposure to radiation as much as possible. Here are some suggestions everyone would be wise to take:

- Avoid unnecessary X-rays.
- Stay at least eight feet away from an operating microwave device.
- Sit at least eight feet away from the television.
- Do not use an electric blanket or heating pad.
- Use an anti-radiation screen on your computer.
- Do not keep a television or computer on the other side of a wall from your bed. Radiation goes through walls.
- Do not live under or near high-power lines.

❖ BIODETOXIFICATION: IN A NUTSHELL

This chart summarizes the various biodetoxification methods and identifies whether you need a professional to provide the remedy.

	Need professional	Do it yourself
Chelation		
Medical	✓	
Herbal/Nutritional		✓†
Exercise		✓ (nonaerobic)
Nutritional therapy	✓*	✓†
Massage		✓
High-heat		✓†
Intestinal cleansing		✓†
Environmental controls		✓

*A professional is necessary if intravenous treatments are required.
†Consultation with a professional is recommended.

Chapter 12

Nutritional Therapies

The second critical component of my treatment cornerstones is nutrition. One of the most fundamental and important ways we can attain and maintain overall health is through what we eat. The saying "garbage in, garbage out" holds very true for the human body: if we fuel our bodies with inferior food and deprive them of sufficient amounts of necessary nutrients, we will suffer the consequences, in the form of illness or even serious disease. The same is true if we are unable to properly process the nutrients we take in, even if they are wholesome and adequate. So for good health, we need both nutritious food and supplements and a properly functioning body to process them correctly.

Although good nutrition is essential for everyone, it is especially important if you have an autoimmune condition. Living with autoimmunity means your body is fighting a difficult and unique battle, because it is fighting itself. So you need to bring in clever reinforcements to subdue the free radicals, eliminate the toxins, and support the healing process.

This chapter explains some of the nutritional strategies I use at the Edelson Center for people with autoimmune disorders. It is important to emphasize that we develop an individual nutritional program for each patient, based on the individual's food sensitivities and preferences, nutritional deficiencies, type and extent of detoxication errors (because various biodetoxification methods deplete the body of different nutrients), and medical conditions that need to be addressed. Thus no two treatment plans are exactly alike.

At the same time, I know that not everyone with an autoimmune disorder or who wishes to follow a biodetoxification program and improve their immune system health comes to the Edelson Center. That's why this chapter also discusses some nutritional strategies for those who want to do what they can at home, preferably with the help of a knowledgeable healthcare professional.

❖ THE BENEFITS OF NUTRITIONAL THERAPY

One reason I stress the need for seeking guidance from a professional is that during biodetoxification, which can take whatever form you choose, toxins are released into the bloodstream and lymph before they are eliminated. Stirring up those metals and chemicals can cause some uncomfortable—but temporary— symptoms, such as headache, nausea, diarrhea, irritability, light-headedness, and fatigue. These symptoms are a natural part of healing from toxicity, but that doesn't mean you need to suffer. That's where nutritional therapy can help. A nutritional diet and conscientious supplementation program can support biodetoxification, reduce and relieve accompanying symptoms, and improve overall health.

❖ NUTRITIONAL THERAPY AND BIODETOXIFICATION

It's not surprising that more people don't seriously equate the state of their health with the quality of food they eat, because most doctors know very little about nutrition and so don't emphasize its importance to their patients. It's also unfortunate that most people don't do something about changing their diet until they are ill. Of course, there is at least one advantage to this: wanting to get well is often a powerful enough incentive to making a positive change in eating habits.

When people with autoimmunity come to me for help, two of the first things they learn about are the importance of biodetoxification, and the role nutrition plays in it. The process of biodetoxification is one of elimination—ridding the body of poisons. During that process—be it chelation, high-temperature sauna, exercise, massage, or colon hydrotherapy—some essential nutrients also leave the body. Biodetoxification is also somewhat traumatic to the body, so nutrients are needed to ease the transition to health.

"I didn't realize how much my food choices affected my health until I got involved in biodetoxification," said Bonnie, a thirty-two-year-old advertising executive who came to me with lupus. She also came with high levels of mercury and various chemicals, including benzene and formaldehyde. What Bonnie learned was that while we were removing toxins from her body, some essential nutrients were going along for the ride and needed to be replaced daily. She also learned that maintaining a balance of nutrients was not only important for biodetoxification to be efficient, but was necessary for fighting free radicals and maintaining good health. "It's probably the best education I ever got on nutrition," she said.

It's an education that I want to share with everyone. That's why patients who undergo biodetoxification receive comprehensive nutritional therapy during treatment at the Center. Generally, nutritional therapy while at the Center includes:

• High doses of selected vitamins, minerals, and other nutrients to replace those lost during biodetoxification, and to facilitate the biodetoxification process. Often we use megadoses, which should only be taken under a doctor's supervision; and intravenous (IV) supplementation, when needed.

• Oils or high-fiber supplements that help the bowels stay regular and efficiently move stool through the intestines.

• Lots of pure water to facilitate the removal of toxins in urine, stool, and sweat, and to help replace the great amount of fluid lost during high-temperature sauna therapy and exercise.

When patients are ready to leave the Center, they are sent home with a nutritional program that has been developed to reflect their specific needs while they continue a reduced detoxification program, one they can follow for the rest of their lives.

Before we get to the supplement and food portion of the program, however, let's look at a critical component of nutritional therapy. The best food in the world will do you little good if your body isn't in shape to process it. One of the biggest problems in the food-processing department, especially among people with autoimmune conditions, is a condition called leaky gut syndrome. It's to that odd-sounding condition that we turn to now.

❖ LEAKY GUT SYNDROME

If you've never heard the phrase "leaky gut syndrome" before, you may be picturing a gut ("gut" is synonymous with bowel or intestine, not stomach) that is dripping out its contents. Actually, you wouldn't be far from the truth. This very common medical condition is characterized by an intestinal lining that is more permeable than normal, which means there are unusually large spaces between the cells that make up the lining. This extra space allows toxic substances such as chemicals, bacteria, viruses, fungi, and large food molecules to "leak out" of the intestines and to enter the bloodstream, where they travel throughout the body. In a healthy gut, these toxins are eliminated.

So what importance does leaky gut have in autoimmunity? Although about one-third of otherwise healthy individuals have leaky gut syndrome (and don't even know it), most people with autoimmunity have this syndrome. The reason leaky gut is nearly always associated with autoimmunity is because chemical toxins and heavy metals, as well as infections, food allergies, and nutritional deficiencies, are present in individuals with autoimmune disorders, and all of these factors are associated with leaky gut syndrome. If you eliminate the factors, you most likely eliminate the leaky gut.

Why the Gut Leaks

Most infectious organisms enter the body through the gastrointestinal (GI) tract, or gut. When the lining of the GI tract is healthy, it performs two basic functions: it allows nutrients from food to pass into the bloodstream, and it prevents invaders such as bacteria, toxins (which create free radicals), and peptides (which lead to allergies and sensitivities) from entering the bloodstream.

Sometimes the lining of the gut becomes damaged—from things like heavy metals, pesticides and other toxic chemicals, bacteria, NSAIDs, fungi, alcohol, and antibiotics—and large pores or spaces form in the walls of the intestines. These holes are like sieves that allow toxic substances to enter the bloodstream. This condition is known as leaky gut syndrome, or intestinal permeability. Once the toxins enter the bloodstream, they may or may not be eliminated from the body, depending on the ability of the liver to perform its detoxication process. If the liver is overloaded with the processing of toxins or is hindered for other reasons, the toxins are dumped back into the bloodstream. In people who are susceptible to autoimmunity, the toxins that are racing through the bloodstream can cause free-radical damage and trigger autoimmunity.

Other problems can occur as well. A secondary effect of a damaged intestinal tract is malabsorption of nutrients, which then leads to nutritional deficiencies. Such deficiencies are clearly detrimental in people who are combating autoimmunity (see box, "Recognizing and Treating Malabsorption," on p. 273).

Symptoms often experienced by people with autoimmunity—fatigue, joint pain, fever, muscle pain, diarrhea, rash, memory deficit, shortness of breath, and others—can be collectively identified as the syndrome known as leaky gut. However, not everyone who has leaky gut has autoimmunity, and vice versa. Also, about one-third of people with leaky gut are asymptomatic (without symptoms).

Healing Leaky Gut Syndrome

Several nutrients are helpful in restoring the integrity of the GI tract. They include:

• Glutamine. This is the main ingredient that the intestinal cells use to maintain and repair the intestinal lining.

• *Lactobacillus gg* and *Lactobacillus plantarum*. These friendly bacteria, or probiotics, help counteract the effects of bad organisms, especially the yeast candida. They also help modulate the immune system. See "The Power of Probiotics," below.

• N-acetylglucosamine (NAG). This nutrient facilitates healing of the intestinal lining and also helps prevent inflammation.

• Nutrients. The antioxidants vitamins C and E, plus lipoic acid and zinc, protect the intestinal lining from free-radical damage.

• Cat's claw (*Uncaria tomentosa*). This herb cleanses the intestinal tract and helps people who have Crohn's disease, leaky gut syndrome, and candidiasis.

• Slippery elm (*Ulmas fulva*). The benefits of this herb are its soothing effect on the GI lining and its stimulation of the secretion of mucus, which protects against the formation of ulcers.

The Power of Probiotics

If "antibiotics" are substances that work against (are destructive to) life, then "probiotics" are for life. And that's exactly why probiotics are used to promote good GI health: they favor the growth of good bacteria in the body.

More than five hundred different species of bacteria live in the intestinal tract. Maintaining a healthy balance of "bad" versus "good" bacteria can be an especially difficult task for people who have autoimmunity and leaky gut syndrome. That's why probiotics are important for people who have autoimmune conditions, as they can help restore the population of good bacteria to the intestinal tract and thus the health of the gut.

There are other reasons why you should consider taking probiotics. If you have an autoimmune disease and are being treated with prednisone, cortisone, or other steroids, or you are taking antibiotics, these drugs are destroying the beneficial bacteria in your GI tract. That means that, instead of these drugs helping you, they can actually cause more problems—namely, leaky gut syndrome and systemic problems such as food allergies and sensitivities.

Certain probiotics are not effective because they are killed by the stomach acid and/or the alkalinity of the small intestine before they reach the colon. The only two that get through to the colon are *Lactobacillus gg* and *Lactobacillus plantarum*. These species have protective mechanisms for those hostile environments. (*Lactobacillus acidophilus* is effective if given as an enema, because then it does not have to get past the stomach acid or alkalinity of the small intestine.)

Recognizing and Treating Malabsorption

Malabsorption is an alteration in the ability of the intestinal tract to absorb nutrients into the bloodstream. (It can also be caused by toxins, food allergies, inflammation, or infection, all common among people with autoimmunity, as well as by radiation or use of antibiotics. That's why many people with autoimmune conditions have malabsorption.) People with malabsorption may have a healthy appetite, but because they are unable to absorb the nutrients from their food, they are often hungry. Malabsorption can also be associated with many other symptoms, depending on the severity of the nutritional deficiencies. They include:

- Diarrhea, sometimes explosive, with foul-smelling stools
- Steatorrhea (excessive fat in the stools)
- Abdominal cramping, bloating, and gas caused by poor carbohydrate and water absorption

- Edema (fluid retention in the tissues) caused by poor protein absorption
- Weight loss and malnutrition caused by an inability to properly absorb protein, carbohydrates, fat, and nutrients
- Muscle cramping caused by low levels of calcium, potassium, and vitamin D
- Irregular heartbeat, caused by low levels of electrolytes (potassium, sodium, and other nutrients responsible for healthy heart functioning)
- Muscle atrophy, due to decreased protein absorption and metabolism

Treatment of malabsorption is designed to heal the gastrointestinal lining and can include glutamine, aloe vera, probiotics, elimination of infections, identification and elimination of allergic foods, removal of toxins, and a comprehensive nutritional program that includes antioxidants and other supplements to bring the individual's nutrient levels up to normal range.

❖ ANTIOXIDANT THERAPY

One of the most powerful defenses we have against the oxidation process caused by free-radical destruction is antioxidants. These substances deactivate free radicals, those villains of autoimmunity. Antioxidants are especially needed by the liver so it can effectively protect the detoxification process (see chapter 11). Although antioxidants are good for everyone, they are especially critical for people who have autoimmune conditions, which is why I initiate aggressive antioxidant therapy—often combining intravenous and oral supplementation—for all my autoimmune patients.

If you have an autoimmune disorder and want to know what steps you can take, or if you just want to prevent possible problems or achieve and maintain a healthy immune system, we also discuss a less aggressive antioxidant program for you at home.

What Are Antioxidants?

Antioxidants can be divided into two categories: natural (not digestive) enzymes, and nutrient-derived antioxidants. In the first category are some names that may be new to you, yet they are your body's first line of antioxidant defense. Some of them are catalase, peroxidase, and superoxide dismutase (SOD). Nutrient-derived antioxidants include vitamin A (retinol), beta-carotene, vitamins C and E, selenium, some of the amino acids, and glutathione.

Getting antioxidants by eating foods such as fruits, vegetables, and whole grains is the best way to supply your body with these important substances. However, supplements are necessary in today's toxic world, because we are constantly being assaulted by chemical toxins and heavy metals that lead to the production of free radicals in our bodies. We need the added protection that antioxidant supplements can give us. Thus for people with autoimmunity, supplementation is especially critical, both during biodetoxification and in the healing process.

How Antioxidants Work

Free radicals, which are highly unstable molecules, are always on the lookout for an electron from another molecule. Once a free radical steals an electron, the "victim" molecule becomes a free radical, which leads to creation of more free radicals. Free radicals are highly destructive molecules, causing damage to cell membranes, DNA, mitochondria, and enzyme functioning, to name just a few effects.

An antioxidant is a molecule that has a full electron saturation in its outer ring. When one of the electrons is pulled off by a free radical, the antioxidant becomes a free radical and grabs an electron from another molecule. As you can see, this action goes on and on until enough antioxidants step in and stop the damaging action from continuing. To do that, you need to ingest the full spectrum of antioxidants, not just one or two. If you take a large amount of just one, like vitamin C, and no others, you actually cause more harm to yourself than good. That's because there aren't enough of the other antioxidants, like vitamin E and beta-carotene, to carry the electrons from one antioxidant to another and into the energy cycle to make energy for the body. Therefore, antioxidants are effective at combating free radicals only if you take a sufficient amount and a wide variety of them . . . and you have enough antioxidant "helpers," too (see "Antioxidant 'Helpers' ").

Critical Antioxidants

The following antioxidants are especially helpful in fighting free-radical damage and are among those I usually prescribe for patients who have an autoimmune condition. Dosages given during intense biodetoxification at the Edelson Center are often mega-doses and are given under medical supervision. Before you embark on any type of supplement program, you should consult with a physician who is knowledgeable about nutrition.

• **Beta-carotene** is a water-soluble antioxidant that is also known as pro-vitamin A, because the liver uses it to create vitamin A. Beta-carotene supplementation is preferred over taking vitamin A (retinol), as the latter can reach toxic levels in the body and cause liver damage. Beta-carotene has the ability to stop the oxidation process and to neutralize toxins found in cigarette smoke, air pollutants, and other environmental toxins. It is especially useful during phase 1 liver detoxication.

• **Vitamin C** is another water-soluble nutrient. The presence of toxins in the body increases the amount of vitamin C that is excreted in the urine, so high doses of this antioxidant are needed daily. Vitamin C also enhances the activity of another antioxidant, glutathione. Vitamin C is recommended during treatment with DMPS, as it accelerates the detoxication process.

• **Vitamin E** is a fat-soluble nutrient that helps protect lipid (fat) cell membranes from oxidative damage. It is especially needed during phase 1 liver detoxication.

• **Selenium** is a mineral that is both an antioxidant and an antioxidant "helper," because it is essential for the activity of glutathione (see "Glutathione," below). It is especially needed during phase 1 liver detoxication. Supplementation of selenium is especially important because our diets are low in this mineral due to crops being grown in selenium-deficient soil.

• **Lipoic acid** is an unusual antioxidant in that it can deactivate both fat- and water-soluble free radicals—no other antioxidant can do that. Because it is fat-soluble, it can get into nerve cells and help stop free-radical damage there, which makes it an especially important antioxidant for people who have MS and other demyelinating disorders. Lipoic acid also raises levels of glutathione.

• **Coenzyme Q10** is an antioxidant and, by definition, a substance that helps enzymes perform their biological chemical reactions. What's special about coenzyme Q10 is that it is needed by every cell in the body in order to produce energy. If you think of each cell as an engine, coenzyme Q10 is the spark that starts the production of energy. If there's no coenzyme Q10, there's no spark and no energy. As an antioxidant, it helps protect the cells against free-radical damage and is found in especially high concentrations in the liver. Remember that the liver is the key organ of biodetoxification (see chapter 11); thus adequate levels of coenzyme Q10 are critical for people who have autoimmunity.

• **Glutathione** and the enzymes that it produces, including glutathione peroxidase, are considered to be the most important antioxidants for overall health and the most powerful fighters of oxidative stress. Glutathione protects against pesticides, plastics, benzene, carbon tetrachloride, heavy metals, cigarette smoke, smog, carbon monoxide, solvents, dyes, phenols, and nitrates by detoxifying these poisons into less toxic forms. This antioxidant and its enzymes are so powerful, in fact, that some scientists believe that in the future we will use a form of glutathione to help clean up the environment. The recommended form is reduced L-glutathione, which is most readily used by the body because it saves the body the energy it takes to reduce it to its active form. It should be taken along with alpha ketoglutaric acid, which helps with the liver detoxification process.

• **Superoxide dismutase** (SOD) is a potent antioxidant, especially against a specific type of free radical called the hydroxyl radical, which Jeffrey Bland, Ph.D., author and authority on nutritional biochemistry, calls the "most toxic free radical." SOD is particulatly important during phase 1 liver detoxication. Although this enzyme is available as an oral and injectable supplement, neither form is useful, because SOD only lasts a few minutes in the body. Unfortunately, food sources of SOD are also ineffective. The body's manufacture of SOD depends on two factors: genetics, which you can do nothing about; and sufficient intake of copper, zinc, and manganese (see the chart at the end of this chapter for recommendations).

Antioxidant "Helpers"

Other nutrients are also needed for liver detoxification to go smoothly. These antioxidant "helpers," or cofactors, include the following:

• **Amino acids.** Several of the amino acids are especially important for treating autoimmunity. Arginine stimulates thymus gland activity. Cysteine is a potent antioxidant; it is needed to make glutathione and is helpful in eliminating heavy metals from the body. Carnitine helps raise energy levels and helps prevent oxidation. I prescribe amino acids depending on the individual's amino acid analysis. Amino acid supplements should not be taken without first consulting your physician.

• **B vitamins** (thiamin, riboflavin, niacin, pantothenate, pyridoxine, and B_{12}). Niacin helps reduce fat levels and so facilitates the elimination of toxins stored in fatty tissue, as are many chemical toxins. Riboflavin and niacin are especially needed during phase 1 liver detoxication. Pyridoxine plays a key role in the production of protein and nucleic acid, both of which are needed by the immune system. Pantothenate stimulates cells of the immune system. All of the B vitamins are involved in mitochondrial (energy production) function.

• **Calcium d-glucarate** is a natural ingredient found in some fruits and vegetables. It assists in the elimination of toxins and helps in phase 2 liver detoxication.

• **Catalase** is an enzyme that speeds up the breakdown of hydrogen peroxide to water and oxygen; thus it is essential for the detoxication process and as an antioxidant.

- **Copper** is a cofactor for catalase and peroxidase and is also critical for SOD production.
- **Glutamine** helps maintain the integrity of the GI mucosal lining and is a major player in phase 2 liver detoxication.
- **Glutathione peroxidase** is one of the most important antioxidant enzymes. It's necessary for intracellular respiration, and thus is critical for the detoxication process, and it also breaks down hydrogen peroxide.
- **Magnesium** has many functions in the body, and indirectly helps fight free radicals.
- **Manganese** is involved in enzyme reactions involving cholesterol and fatty acid synthesis. It is especially needed during phase 1 liver detoxication, and is also critical for production of SOD.
- **Molybdenum** is a trace mineral that is needed for phase 1 liver detoxication,
- **N-acetylcysteine** is a precursor to glutathione. It is especially needed during phase 2 liver detoxication.
- **Zinc** is involved in phase 1 liver detoxication and is a cofactor for many enzyme activities. It is also crucial for SOD production.

❖ A GOOD AUTOIMMUNE (AND ALL-ROUND) DIET

Three or more times a day, every day, you have the chance to help your body by providing it with food that not only promotes the detoxication process but also enhances overall health and does not add more toxins to the body. It is unfortunate that most doctors in the United States have little or no training in nutritional biochemistry; this deficiency has contributed to the ignorance of many people about the critical impact food has on their health.

When a person has an autoimmune condition, nutrition becomes of paramount importance. In fact, food can be a medicine that helps heal and maintain good health. (Individuals also should undergo food allergy and sensitivity testing to identify which foods they should avoid.) A nutritious diet is important both during the biodetoxification process and after the program is complete. Generally, my guidelines for a healthy diet are:

• Eat a varied diet that includes small to moderate portions. Overeating stresses the mitochondria, increases free-radical production, and overburdens the liver, making it more difficult for detoxication to proceed.

• Eat foods that are as chemical-free as possible. (Avoid or significantly reduce intake of processed, refined foods, and choose organic and whole foods when possible.)

• Choose foods that are high in fiber and low in fat: the overall breakdown of the diet should be 60 percent carbohydrates, 20 percent fat, and 20 percent protein.

What do I mean about food being medicine? Take cruciferous vegetables, for example. Broccoli, cauliflower, cabbage, brussels sprouts, and other vegetables in this category enhance phase 1 liver detoxication. That's because these vegetables contain a substance called indole, which triggers detoxication enzymes. Foods that are high in fiber (e.g., whole grains, fruits, vegetables, legumes) are good medicine because they help move toxins out of the body in stool. And what better medicine could you ask for than antioxidants, which are found in abundance in most fruits and vegetables?

Sitting Down at the Table

The following guidelines should be followed for optimum detoxication and for overall health maintenance. In other words, we are presenting you with eating suggestions you can follow for the rest of your life, starting now.

PROTEIN

Protein should make up 20 percent of your daily caloric intake. That means that if the average number of calories you need to maintain your health and weight is 2,000 calories, 400 of those calories should be from protein. Recommended sources include lentils, beans, soy (see "Soy Foods," below), nuts, seeds, fish (deep-sea, cold-water fish only), and organic chicken. Conventionally produced red meat should be avoided because it contains hormones, steroids, antibiotics, bad fats, and the potential for food poisoning. If you do eat red meat, it should be organic and in moderation.

CARBOHYDRATES

This is the largest category—60 percent of your daily intake—and the most versatile. On 2,000 calories per day, carbohydrates should make up 1,200. Healthy carbohydrates include fruits, vegetables, rice, and whole grain breads, pastas, and cereals. When possible, buy organic and whole grain products.

Carbohydrates can be simple or complex. Simple carbohydrates are found in fruits, sugar, and honey. Foods in the complex category include vegetables, grains, and legumes and are excellent sources of fiber and energy. Sugar, as you'll see below (see "Foods to Avoid"), compromises the immune system. Ideally, most of the carbohydrates you eat should be complex, with the minority consisting of fruits.

FATS

Fats are always a touchy category until we understand that there are both good and bad ones. Most fats fall into the latter category. One of them is saturated fats, found in meat, fowl, dairy products, and tropical oils. Besides raising your cholesterol level—and your risk of heart disease, cancer, and other serious conditions—these oils increase the production of prostaglandins, which cause inflammation. Polyunsaturated fat, found in most prepackaged foods, is a rancid, free-radical-creating fat. Other free-radical builders include trans fatty acids and hydrogenated fats.

Good fats include essential fatty acids, which are important for people with autoimmunity (see "Essential Fatty Acids," on page 289), and monounsaturated fats. Moderate amounts of nuts, seeds, avocados, olive oil, olives, flaxseed oil, nut oils, fatty fish, and blackcurrant and evening primrose oils can provide you with healthy fats, which should make up no more than 20 percent of your daily caloric intake. Generally, it is best to include lots of organic, low-fat foods such as fruits, vegetables, legumes, and whole grains in your diet, and eliminate fried foods. Red meat, fowl, dairy products, and eggs are okay if they are organic and consumed in moderation.

FRUITS AND VEGETABLES: ANTIOXIDANT POWER

Less than 10 percent of Americans eat the recommended daily five to nine servings of fruits and vegetables (see "How Much Is a Serving?" on p. 289). Yet these foods are our best sources of vitamins, minerals, antioxidants, and fiber (see "Food Sources of Essential Nutrients," on p. 288). To avoid toxins, organic produce is recommended over conventionally grown fruits and vegetables.

FIBER

Fiber plays a critical role in detoxication because it helps rid the body of toxins through the feces and regulates bowel function. The recommended daily intake of fiber is 20 to 35 grams, yet most Americans eat only about 11 grams. Why? Because the typical American diet consists of a lot of meat, fowl, and dairy—all of which contain no fiber. To get the recommended amount of fiber into your diet, you need to include plenty of vegetables, whole grains, fruits, beans, and legumes (see box, "High-Fiber Foods," on p. 287).

SOY FOODS

Soybeans and foods made from them, including tofu, texturized vegetable protein, soy milk, tempeh, miso, and tamari, are recognized for their antioxidant powers and cancer-fighting abilities. They are also an excellent source of protein (and a good substitute for red meat as long as you have a source of B_{12}; supplement if necessary) and also contain fiber while being low in fat. Imitation meat and dairy products made from soy—including soy dogs, burgers, bacon, ham, turkey, and cheeses—are now available in mainstream supermarkets across the country. Make sure the soybeans and the foods made from them are organic. (Note: some people are allergic or sensitive to soy. Allergy testing is recommended if you suspect you have such a condition.)

LEGUMES

Legumes—beans, lentils, and split peas, all organic—are an excellent source of protein, complex carbohydrates, fiber, vitamins, and minerals. And they are low in fat, so these versatile foods seem to have it all. They can serve as a meat substitute and should be included as part of a healthy diet.

WHOLE GRAINS AND CEREALS

Organic whole grains are an excellent source of most B vitamins—which are essential for aiding the liver in the detoxication process—and several other antioxidants. They are rich in complex carbohydrates, vitamin E, fiber, protein, and other necessary nutrients.

Most people think of wheat when they hear the words "whole grains," but there are many more from which to choose, which is especially helpful if you are allergic or sensitive to wheat. Try amaranth, barley, couscous, brown rice, buckwheat, kamut, millet, and quinoa. Most of these are readily available in mainstream supermarkets.

FOODS TO AVOID

Some food substances are better off rarely passing through your lips, especially if you have an autoimmune disorder. Eliminating these items from your diet as much as possible can make a significant difference in your health.

• **Sugar.** Consuming more than 100 grams of sugar daily can reduce the body's ability to fight infection, overburden the adrenal glands and pancreas, promote bone loss, and deplete the body of B vitamins, vitamin C, and minerals. Yet the average American eats about 150 grams of sugar daily, setting up a not-so-sweet road to medical problems, including chronic fatigue, candidiasis, and nutritional deficiencies. Sugar is hidden in many foods, so read labels carefully. Cereals, baked goods, diet items (they may be low-fat, but manufacturers add more sugar to pump up the taste), candy, condiments, and packaged mixes are some of the biggest offenders.

• **Alcohol.** A little alcohol—one or two drinks per day—appears to be okay for healthy individuals, but even small amounts are not recommended if you have an autoimmune disorder. Alcohol hinders efficient liver detoxication, reduces the ability of lymphocytes to fight infection, causes fatigue and muscle weakness, depletes the body of zinc, magnesium, manganese, vitamin C, and the B vitamins, and causes cell death.

• **Caffeine.** Americans love caffeine, but we would be better off without this legal drug. The caffeine in coffee, tea, cola, and aspirin can stress the adrenal glands and interfere with mineral absorption.

• **Cow milk products.** Cow's milk and products made from it can be problematic for several reasons. The biggest problem is that many people are allergic to dairy products. Another is lactose intolerance, which means individuals cannot process the milk sugar (lactose) found in cow's milk. Yet another reason for avoiding milk products is the presence of additives in milk (see the item "Food additives," below). Alternatives to milk products include soy milk, rice milk, and nut milks, with cheeses, frozen desserts, and yogurts made from these products, so you can still enjoy a pizza made with soy cheese, chocolate soy milk, and fruit-flavored soy yogurt.

• **Food additives.** More than 2,800 substances can legally be added to our food. Included in this list are various preservatives, artificial colorings and flavorings, and other chemicals. Some of them, such as monosodium glutamate (MSG), nitrates, nitrites, and various food dyes, are known to cause allergic reactions in some individuals, as well as disturb liver and kidney function and destroy cells. Therefore, it is important to avoid processed foods as much as possible. Instead, focus on whole grains and beans and organically grown fruits and vegetables.

• **Hormones and drugs.** Cows, pigs, chickens, and other food animals are routinely fed or injected with synthetic hormones, steroids, antibiotics, and other drugs in order to fatten them up faster and to disguise signs of disease. Even fish, many of which are now "grown" on fish farms, are given antibiotics to fight disease. In fact, approximately 75 percent of the antibiotics produced in North America are given to food animals. These antibiotics and other substances can then be passed along to the people who eat these animals. Antibiotic-resistant bacteria that develop in these animals can also be transferred to humans. Organically raised, free-range meats are available; but better yet, skip the saturated fat and cholesterol and turn to other protein sources (see "Protein," on p. 282).

High-Fiber Foods

Food	Portion	Fiber
Fiber One Cereal	½ cup	10 g
Prunes, cooked	½ cup	10 g
Bran Chex	½ cup	9 g
Lentils, cooked	½ cup	8 g
Kidney beans, cooked	½ cup	8 g
Broccoli, fresh, cooked	½ cup	7 g
Sweet potato, baked	1 small	7 g
Pita, whole wheat	1	7 g
Refried beans	½ cup	6 g
Corn, kernels	½ cup	5 g
Pasta, whole wheat	1 cup	5 g
Pear	1 medium	5 g
Beets, pickled	½ cup	4 g
Apple, with peel	1 medium	4 g
Peas, green, cooked	½ cup	4 g
Sauerkraut, canned	½ cup	4 g
Orange	1 medium	4 g
Cantaloupe	1 cup	3 g
Spinach, cooked	½ cup	3 g
Cauliflower, cooked	1 cup	3 g
Carrots, cooked	½ cup	2 g
Rice, brown	½ cup	2 g

Food Sources of Essential Nutrients

The best way to get your antioxidants and other essential nutrients is to eat them, and there is no shortage of options. Here are just a few of the richest sources of some common nutrients.

- **Beta-carotene:** apricots, broccoli, cantaloupe, carrots, kale, pumpkin, spinach, squash
- **Vitamin B$_1$:** brewer's yeast (avoid if you have candida infection), brown rice, chickpeas, navy beans, soybeans, wheat germ, whole grain flour
- **Vitamin B$_2$:** almonds, black-eyed peas, brewer's yeast, wheat germ
- **Vitamin B$_3$:** beets, brewer's yeast, peanuts, sunflower seeds
- **Vitamin B$_5$:** brewer's yeast, corn, lentils, peanuts, peas, soybeans, sunflower seeds, wheat germ, whole grain flour
- **Vitamin B$_6$:** avocados, bananas, brewer's yeast, brown rice, carrots, lentils, soybeans, sunflower seeds, wheat germ, whole grain flour
- **Vitamin B$_{12}$:** meat, B$_{12}$-enriched cereals and soy products such as soy milk, tofu, and miso
- **Vitamin C:** blueberries, broccoli, brussels sprouts, cabbage, grapefruit, guava, kale, lemons, oranges, peppers, potatoes, spinach, strawberries, tomatoes
- **Vitamin E:** almonds, filberts, oils (olive, peanut, wheat germ), walnuts, wheat germ, whole grain flour

- **Folic acid:** barley, brewer's yeast, brown rice, most fruits, green leafy vegetables, lentils, oranges, peas, soybeans, sprouts, wheat germ
- **Copper:** barley, blackstrap molasses, lentils, mushrooms, oatmeal, nuts, peanuts, wheat germ
- **Magnesium:** barley, broccoli, cantaloupe, carrots, millet, onions, parsley, pecans, spinach, tomatoes
- **Selenium:** barley, broccoli, cabbage, celery, cucumbers, garlic, mushrooms, onions, wheat and rice bran, whole grain flour
- **Zinc:** mushrooms, soybeans, sunflower seeds, wheat germ, whole grain flour
- **Coenzyme Q10:** peanuts, spinach

How Much Is a Serving of Fruits and Vegetables?

One serving equals any one of the following:

½ cup cooked or chopped raw fruit or vegetable
1 cup raw leafy vegetable
1 medium piece of fruit
¼ cup dried fruit
6 ounces vegetable or fruit juice

❖ ESSENTIAL FATTY ACIDS

Essential fatty acids (EFAs) are substances that perform many functions in the body—among them, keeping the immune system functioning properly and maintaining blood vessel health. These fatty acids fall into two general categories: omega-3 and omega-6. Examples of omega-3 EFAs include EPA (eicosapentaenoic acid) and DHA (docosahexaenoic acid), which are found in fish oils and some vegetable oils; and alpha-linolenic acid, which is found especially in flaxseed oil (also known as linseed oil). Examples of omega-6 oils include linoleic acid and gamma-linolenic acid (GLA). Most omega-6 EFAs are found in animal products and contribute to inflammation (linoleic acid), but one, GLA, is found in plants and prevents inflammation. This EFA is found in evening primrose oil, borage oil, and blackcurrant oil and is usually taken as a supplement.

All of these essential fatty acids—EPA, DHA, and GLA—are precursors of prostaglandins, such as PG1, which have anti-inflammatory and anti-autoimmune effects. They also reduce the activity of the prostaglandins (such as PG2) that promote inflammation. This ability to *modulate* inflammation is what makes EFAs an essential part of immunotherapy.

Maintaining a proper balance between omega-3 and omega-6 EFAs is critical to good health and to eliminating inflammation. Unfortunately, achieving and keeping that balance through diet isn't always easy to do, because Americans tend to consume much more omega-6s (in animal foods) than omega-3s. One way to get a better balance is to take an omega-3 supplement and limit your intake of animal products.

What Makes Essential Fatty Acids So Good?

Essential fatty acids are different from other fats (e.g., saturated fats like those found in meat and cheese) in molecular structure, and that physical difference—too complex to discuss here—is part of what makes them good. They're also beneficial because they perform many essential roles in the body. For example, they:

- Supply the raw materials needed to make prostaglandins, substances that are important for reduction of pain and inflammation
- Help fight infections, bacteria, and yeast, problems that plague many people who have autoimmunity
- Are needed for the body's production of tumor necrosis factor, also important in fighting autoimmunity
- Store energy, which is particularly helpful for people who suffer with fatigue
- Are needed for building cells and membranes, necessary for the healing process
- Support brain health; DHA is the most important molecule for this function

Who Needs EFAs?

Experts believe that approximately 80 percent of Americans are deficient in EFAs. This presents a serious health threat, especially when you consider that they help protect against more than sixty health conditions, including autoimmune disorders, heart disease, cancer, and skin disease. People who have rheumatoid arthritis and lupus often report much improvement in their level of pain and inflammation when they take EFAs.

EFAs and Rheumatoid Arthritis

In 2000, a review of nearly forty research papers on the therapeutic use of gamma-linolenic acid (GLA) revealed that this essential fatty acid appears to be an important part of the diet for people who have rheumatoid arthri-

---

tis. Dr. Marya Zilberberg, of Metaworks Inc., in Medford, Massachusetts, who headed the research, noted that GLA consistently reduces joint stiffness and inflammation and does not cause any serious side effects. In particular, Dr. Zilberberg found that GLA reduces morning stiffness by 60 to 65 percent, a significant problem for people with rheumatoid arthritis, and one problem that many patients view as the most debilitating part of their disease.

How to Get Your EFAs

The easiest and most effective way to get your EFAs is to take flaxseed oil, preferably organic and unrefined. Flaxseed oil is unique because it contains both omega-3 and omega-6 fatty acids in good amounts. In fact, flaxseed oil is the richest source of omega-3 fatty acids—it contains more than twice the amount of omega-3 fatty acids found in fish oils, another source of omega-3s (see below). Because flaxseed oil is easily damaged by heat and light, you don't want to cook with it. Instead, add 1 to 2 tablespoons of oil to your food each day. Sprinkle it over your salad or vegetables; drizzle it on your mashed potatoes or garlic toast (after removing the bread from the oven); make a salad dressing with it (see box, "Using Flaxseed Oil," below). You can also blend it into a smoothie, some applesauce, or even take it by the spoonful, but it's not too palatable that way.

A downside of flaxseed oil is that to make EPA and DHA from flax, the body needs a special enzyme. Many people with chronic disease lack this enzyme (your doctor can test for this deficiency), so if you are among those who don't have it, you may need to take fish oil instead.

Another EFA that helps eliminate inflammation is GLA. The best sources are evening primrose oil, blackcurrant oil, and borage oil, all available in health food stores and pharmacies. Consult with a knowledgeable physician to determine the best dosages for you. Results are not immediate; it can take up to three months for significant changes to take place, although most people notice some benefit before then.

Tamara noticed improvement in the amount of inflammation and pain from rheumatoid arthritis after taking EFAs for only eight weeks. "I'm taking one tablespoon of flaxseed oil daily, plus 1000 mg evening primrose oil," she says. "I can get out of bed much more easily in the morning, I don't have stiffness like I used to, and my pain has been cut in half." She also noted some other benefits. "My eczema is gone," she said. "And my skin isn't dry anymore; it looks better than it has in twenty years."

Along with taking supplements of EFA, Tamara and others who have autoimmune conditions can expect best results if they significantly limit their intake of saturated fats, which are found in animal products.

Fishy EFAs: Are They Safe?

Some health professionals recommend eating fish or taking fish oil (EPA and DHA) supplements to get your EFAs. Only oily fish— for example, sardines, salmon, mackerel, herring, and tuna—have adequate amounts of EFAs. Eating oily fish two or three times a week can provide you with a good dose of EFAs, but many people don't like fish or object to eating it on ethical grounds. Fish oil capsules are available in health food stores; however, it isn't clear whether they provide the same benefits as you could get from eating the fish. Also, given the high levels of contamination (mercury and other metals) in most fish, the oils may be similarly contaminated. Some companies, however, have analyzed their oil capsules and have found them to be safe (see the appendix).

Using Flaxseed Oil

3 tbsp red wine
1½ tbsp extra-virgin olive oil
1½ tbsp flaxseed oil
2 cloves garlic, minced
2 tbsp minced fresh parsley
½ tsp sea salt
2 tbsp finely ground flaxseeds
1 tbsp Dijon mustard

Combine all ingredients and shake well. Serves 2.

When you bring your flaxseed oil home, keep it refrigerated in a dark glass bottle. Use it within two months, or you can freeze it for up to one year. Never heat it. If it turns rancid, throw it out. Once the oil is damaged, toxic molecules called lipid peroxides form.

❖ PANCREATIC ENZYMES

As food leaves the stomach and enters the small intestine, enzymes are needed to help continue the digestive process. Those enzymes—among them lipase, trypsin, and amylase—come from the pancreas, a small organ that lies close to the stomach and liver. In addition to helping with normal digestion, pancreatic enzymes can also help break down food particles so they are not identified as invaders by the immune system.

If the pancreas is unable to produce enough of these enzymes, which can occur because of trauma to the organ or disease, the result can be a problem with digestion, called maldigestion syndrome. Maldigestion is a deficiency in the pancreatic enzymes or small intestinal peptidase enzymes.

Supplements of pancreatic enzymes, either as a pill or a powder that can be sprinkled on food, are available over the counter and should be taken according to package directions.

❖ SUMMARY: BETTER NUTRITION FOR AUTOIMMUNITY

The prescription for treating autoimmunity nutritionally at home is simple: (1) modify your diet to include healthy food, as described above; (2) take supplements to promote immune health, assist detoxication, and enhance overall health (see list below); and (3) take enzymes if it is proved that you need them. I also strongly recommend a fourth item: consult with a professional who is knowledgeable about nutrition and autoimmunity so you can tailor your nutritional program to your specific needs.

Antioxidants and Other Essential Nutrients

The dosages given below are suggestions only. What you need will depend on your diet, overall health, whether you have an autoimmune disorder, and whether you are pursuing a biodetoxification program. (In the case of the last, see chapter 11 for more information on specific supplements.)

Beta-carotene	10,000–30,000 IU
Vitamin C	250–1000 IU
Vitamin E	400–800 IU

Vitamin B_1	10–100 mg
Vitamin B_2	10–100 mg
Vitamin B_3 (niacin/niacinamide)	10–100 mg/10–30 mg*
Vitamin B_5	25–100 mg
Vitamin B_6	25–100 mg
Folic acid	400–800 mcg
Vitamin B_{12}	200–400 mcg
Selenium	100–200 mcg
Boron	1–2 mg
Calcium	800–1500 mg
Copper	1–2 mg
Magnesium	400–750 mg
Manganese	10–15 mg
Molybdenum	500–1000 mcg
Zinc	15–30 mg
Coenzyme Q10	30 mg

*Niacin causes flushing in some people; niacinamide is a no-flush alternative.

Chapter 13

Immunotherapy

As you've seen so far, treating autoimmunity can involve many different healing techniques and approaches. We've talked about two of my three treatment cornerstones: taking things out of the body (biodetoxification) and adding things back into the body (nutritional therapy). Now we're going to show you how to modulate or regulate your immune system using immunotherapy.

Immunotherapy is exactly what it sounds like: therapy designed to nurture and heal the immune system. "Immune modulation" is a phrase often used to explain immunotherapy. The phrase has a soothing ring to it, and indeed, the purpose of immune system modulation is to modulate—harmonize or balance—the immune system. That is, it either stimulates a depressed system or downregulates an overactivated one. For people with autoimmunity, whose immune systems are running on full throttle, immune modulation is just what the doctor ordered. Substances that act as immune system modulators work largely on allergic-type reactions, like inflammation, which is a classic sign in most autoimmune conditions.

In this chapter, we share with you some of the immune modulators I prescribe for my patients. These include, but are not limited to, enzyme potentiated desensitization (EPD), transfer factor, thymus extracts, ozone therapy, human growth hormone, and the hormone DHEA. We also look at a few Chinese herbs that have immune modulation abilities, such as dong quai and ginseng. Some of these modulators can be administered only by a physician; others are available over the counter. If you try immune modulators on your own, consult with your physician before starting them.

❖ TRANSFER FACTOR

In the late 1940s, Dr. H. Sherwood Lawrence discovered various types of molecules that are transferred from mothers to their children through the placenta. These molecules help establish the immune system in newborns. He also found that if you added these molecules, called transfer factors, to an existing immune system, say, in an adult, the ability of the immune system to fight infection and disease would increase dramatically. That happens because the transfer factors "teach" the immune system to recognize specific invaders (bacteria, viruses, fungi) they should be attacking and for which immunity has already been established.

For example, if you have already had the measles, your body created antibodies against the measles virus and so now has a memory of that invader. If you were to be exposed to the measles virus again, your body would recognize it immediately and fight it off before it even had a chance to cause a problem, because immunity had already been established. Transfer factors, which are produced by T-cells, are the key to the immune system's memory of past invaders.

Natural and Unnatural Transfer Factors

If your mother breast-fed you during the first few days of your life, many of the several million natural transfer factors circulating through your body were transferred to you through your mother's colostrum. Colostrum is the first milklike substance that is excreted from all milk-producing mammals—including humans and cows. It is nature's richest source of concentrated transfer factors, and it helps keep an infant healthy while its own immune system is maturing. If you were not breast-fed, your body produced transfer factors, but you may be missing some.

Among people who have an autoimmune disease such as CFIDS, lupus, or MS, pathogens may be a trigger or a cause. Treatment with transfer factors may provide those people with the "missing" molecules they need to destroy the problem pathogens.

For about forty years the only way to get transfer factor was to extract it from blood so it could be made into an injectable solution. This process was extremely expensive, and few people could afford it. Fortunately, in the late 1980s scientists discovered that transfer factor was also found in cow's colostrum. Today, transfer factor is extracted from cow's colostrum using a process that removes all the milk proteins and then extracts the transfer factor so it can be placed into capsules. Removing all the milk proteins is important, as many people are lactose intolerant or are allergic to milk protein.

Treatment with unnatural transfer factor means receiving molecules from bovine colostrum, preferably from healthy, organically fed cows. Bovine colostrum is used because it is available in great quantities and it contains large numbers of various transfer factors. In fact, manufacturers test their product to see that it contains effective levels of each transfer factor. Crossing species and giving cow colostrum to humans has been shown to be safe and effective, although some people object to it on ethical grounds.

Are Transfer Factors for You?

Paula had been diagnosed with CFIDS one year before coming to my Center. At twenty-seven, she was a graduate student in psychology and had reduced her course load because of her fatigue and muscle weakness. We decided to include transfer factors as part of her treatment program because she had a history of Epstein-Barr viral infection and a current infection with the yeast candida. Paula also said that her CFIDS symptoms had started immediately after she had an acute attack of viral bronchitis, which suggested her immune system could benefit from transfer factors.

Paula experienced dramatic improvement after six months of treatment with transfer factors as well as antioxidant therapy, high-temperature sauna for chemical toxicity, and probiotics for her gastrointestinal tract. It's important to remember that transfer factors support immune system functioning and do not "cure" a problem. Thus, transfer factors alone would not have helped Paula significantly, but by the same token, they enhanced the healing process when used along with the other therapies. Whether transfer factors can help you is something you need to discuss with your physician.

Using Transfer Factors

Even though transfer factors derived from cows are more cost-effective than the old method of extracting it from human blood, this therapy is still expensive. Patients typically need at least three to four months of treatment before positive results can be expected, which adds to the expense.

One way to know that transfer factor therapy is working is to experience some side effects. After only a few weeks of treatment, Paula noted some flulike symptoms and a low fever, which continued for about a month. These symptoms are common, because suddenly the immune system is able to recognize and respond to pathogens it was not able to react to previously. This "aha!" factor can result in symptoms like Paula experienced.

Transfer factor supplements are produced by several different manufacturers and are available over the counter. They should be taken according to package directions and with your doctor's supervision. I recommend the latter, not because transfer factor supplements are dangerous, but because they work along with other treatments you may be taking, including medications.

❖ ENZYME POTENTIATED DESENSITIZATION

"I absolutely hate getting shots, but boy, this treatment really works," said Laura as she rolled up her sleeve. The shots she was talking about were enzyme potentiated desensitization (EPD), a method of immunotherapy in which extremely small doses of allergens are injected into people to desensitize them to their allergies. EPD is used successfully to treat food and inhalant allergies as well as chemical sensitivities. (Currently EPD is available in the United States through the Food and Drug Administration's Compassionate Use program, which allows people to engage in non-FDA-approved therapies for individual use only.)

Laura, who has lupus, came to me with sensitivities to dairy products, nuts, wheat, dust mites, cigarette smoke, and terpenes (substances found in natural items such as trees and petrochemicals). After only three treatments, given every eight weeks, she noticed a significant difference in her response to these allergens. Because of the severity of her allergies, she will need as many as twenty treatments, but the length of time between shots will increase now that she has responded to the first few.

What Is Enzyme Potentiated Desensitization?

In the 1960s, Dr. Leonard McEwen in Britain was trying to find a treatment for nasal polyps when he stumbled upon a way to eliminate nasal allergies. (Unfortunately, the polyps remained.) It seems that the enzyme hyaluronidase, which he was using to eliminate nasal polyps, contains a contaminant enzyme called beta-glucuronidase. Dr. McEwen discovered that the use of beta-glucuronidase, along with very low doses of allergens, resulted in desensitization to the allergens.

EPD soon became a standard way to treat allergies in the United Kingdom. After all, beta-glucuronidase is found naturally in the body, so introducing more of it in an injection is safe. EPD is proven to be very effective, especially for people who have severe allergies. It does require a commitment on the part of patients to be very careful about their exposure to allergens during their treatment. Because treatment can take up to a year or longer, some people decide they will try to avoid all contact with all their allergens. But that task can be overwhelming for many people who have severe allergies or who can't avoid contact with some of the allergens in their environment.

How Does EPD Work?

Each EPD treatment consists of one shot that contains two ingredients: a minute amount of various allergens, and a small amount of beta-glucuronidase. The shot is given in the forearm area just under the top layer of the skin (intradermal injection). The goal of this treatment is to build resistance in the immune system to the substances to which the individual is sensitive, such as lactose (in dairy products), gluten (in wheat), and terpenes.

Scientists believe EPD works by increasing the production of T8 suppressor lymphocytes (a type of immune system cell). One job of T8 cells is to regulate the action of T4 cells, which are responsible for allergic reactions. In people who have allergies, T8 suppressor action is poor, thus allowing T4 cells to run rampant.

The EPD method has been under intense investigation since 1993 in an ongoing study in the United States (see box, "EPD: Where Are We Now?" below). In 1996, it was reported that 85 percent of the people being treated stopped after sixteen to eighteen shots because they had no recurrence of symptoms. One benefit of EPD is that if symptoms should return at any time after they have disappeared, a booster treatment will return you to a symptom-free existence.

What's It Like to Take EPD?

For several days before and after receiving EPD treatment, patients should avoid various allergenic substances, such as perfumes, tobacco smoke, dust, pets, caffeine, and body lotions, as individuals can become more sensitized to these items if they are present when treatment is given. They are also advised to avoid excessive physical stress, such as using a sauna, sexual activity, or hard exercise. These and other suggested restrictions are explained in what is commonly referred to as the "pink book," instructions published by the American EPD Society for people who are undergoing the treatment. Your doctor will discuss the restrictions with you.

The EPD treatment program can be approached in two ways:

simple or complex. People with autoimmune conditions nearly always need the complex approach, which requires many more injections than the simple method that is usually reserved for people who have seasonal allergies. Severe conditions, such as lupus, rheumatoid arthritis, or other autoimmune disorders, usually require twenty or more treatments. While the first few shots may be given about eight weeks apart, the length of time between shots gradually increases until a year or more can pass between treatments. This makes treatments little more than a minor inconvenience.

EPD: Where Are We Now?

As of July 2001, more than 120 doctors had participated in the eight years of study of EPD, and more than 10,000 patients had received in excess of 58,000 doses of the immunotherapy. It did not, however, have the approval of the Food and Drug Administration. Then, in November 2001, the FDA's Compassionate Use rule went into effect. This mandate allows individuals to use therapies not approved by the FDA for their own personal use. Because EPD is now considered to be an experimental treatment, insurance companies do not cover the costs. However, once the data from the study are released, it is hoped that EPD will be viewed as a credible form of treatment and will be covered by at least some insurance providers. Outside the United States, EPD treatments are available in Canada, the United Kingdom, Italy, and a few other countries.

How Effective Is EPD?

Between 80 and 90 percent of people who undergo EPD get significant relief, although some people may feel worse for a while before they feel better. This is not unusual: after all, the body is learning how to react and adjust to many foreign substances all at the same time. However, about 60 percent of patients have a good response to their first injection, and after three doses, most people notice some improvement. Conditions that have been treated successfully include chemical sensitivities, food allergies, preservative allergies, Crohn's disease, ulcerative colitis, rheumatoid arthritis, ankylosing spondylitis, and lupus.

❖ THYMUS EXTRACTS

The thymus gland is the kingpin of the immune system because it produces T-cells (see chapter 1) and several hormones that regulate many immune functions. When levels of these hormones or T-cells are low in the blood, people have an increased susceptibility to infection. The thymus is also highly susceptible to damage from free radicals, thus damage to this gland is especially evident in people who have autoimmune disorders.

How Thymus Extracts Work

One way to improve functioning of the thymus gland and treat autoimmunity is to take thymus glandular extracts. Glandular therapy is based on the homeopathic principle of "like cures like." The concept is that organ cells from an animal will strengthen the same gland or organ in people. In this case, people take thymus gland extract, which is derived from the thymus gland of young calves, with the hope that it will stimulate thymus function and the production of hormones and T-cells. These extracts are available over the counter in capsule form, and via injection from physicians. The suggested daily dose should be equivalent to 120 mg pure polypeptides.

Treating Erin

Thymus extracts were one of the treatments I prescribed for Erin, a twenty-nine-year-old marketing representative who came to me with chronic fatigue and immunodeficiency syndrome (CFIDS), a persistent candida infection, hay fever, and severe food allergies. As part of her treatment program we chose oral (capsules) thymus extract because it can boost production of T-cells, which help fight infections such as candida as well as certain bacteria, fungi, and viruses. It can also improve the symptoms of hay fever and food allergies when it's used along with an elimination diet, which Erin agreed to try. Erin also began antioxidant therapy, as these nutrients, plus zinc, can help restore thymus activity (see chapter 12). After only three weeks, Erin noticed an improvement in her level of fatigue and weakness. By the fourth month of treatment, Erin's hay fever symptoms and candida infection had disappeared, and her food allergy symptoms were much improved. Naturally, her improvement was not solely the result of taking thymus extracts, but they were an essential part of the whole treatment plan.

Are Thymus Extracts Safe?

No side effects have been definitely associated with the use of thymus extracts. However, it is important that you purchase these products from reputable companies, because if the material has not been processed properly, the elements (enzymes, vitamins, minerals, hormone precursors, and other factors in thymus extract) will not be active and be of benefit.

One cautionary note: thymus extracts are dietary supplements and therefore are not regulated by the same strict governmental guidelines that regulate drugs. We mention this because of the risk of mad cow disease. Although bans have been placed on the importation of cow glands from countries where mad cow disease has been found, the ban does not extend to supplements. Therefore, theoretically there is a risk of mad cow disease from thymus extracts. Contact the manufacturer of the supplement and inquire about the source of the extract. Domestic (versus imported) sources are believed to be safe. Generally, it is up to you to decide how real the risk is to you, and to get your doctor's approval before taking the extract.

❖ DHEA

Dehydroepiandrosterone (DHEA) may be best known as an "anti-aging" hormone. Because it's been shown that levels of DHEA decline steadily and rapidly as we age, some people take the supplement to slow down the aging process.

We're interested in DHEA because it's long been known that it can suppress the immune system. Thus it can help some people who have autoimmunity conditions, and has been especially beneficial for those who have rheumatoid arthritis or lupus. It also can reduce allergic reactions.

DHEA is produced by the adrenal glands and is considered to be the mother of hormones, because it is eventually converted into other hormones, such as estrogen, progesterone, and testosterone. Because it is a hormone and is capable of having a significant impact on bodily functions, we are careful when we use it as a supplement. That means I only prescribe dosages that will bring an individual's DHEA level up to his or her normal range. That also means it is necessary to know your range *right now* before you can know how much DHEA to take. Therefore, I strongly recommend that you consult with a professional knowledgeable about DHEA before you start to take it, and that you have a blood test taken periodically to monitor your DHEA levels.

Although some scientists argue that not enough research has been done to identify the benefits and risks of normalizing DHEA levels in individuals, I find that the benefits are significant in many of my patients. Minor side effects may include acne, unwanted body hair in women (usually on the face), mood swings, and insomnia. DHEA supplements should always be taken with a small amount of food that contains fat (e.g., peanut butter, avocado) to aid absorption.

❖ OZONE THERAPY

Millions of people in countries all over the world benefit from a medical treatment that is effective in cases of autoimmune disorders and acute infections. In Germany alone, more than twelve million people with chronic illnesses have been treated since World War II. Although some physicians in the United States consider it to be experimental, twelve states have passed laws that allow physicians to administer it. The name of this treatment is ozone therapy.

"When I first heard about ozone therapy, I thought to myself, isn't ozone dangerous?" said Chantel, a thirty-two-year-old art museum curator who came to me with a diagnosis of lupus. "I mean, aren't we always being warned about the hole in the ozone layer? So I didn't understand at first how and why ozone therapy could help me."

Ozone is a form of oxygen that has an extra atom (O_3), which makes it heavier than regular oxygen (O_2). It is produced when ultraviolet light from the sun irradiates oxygen in the air or, to make ozone for therapeutic purposes, when medical-grade oxygen is passed through an energy field created by ultraviolet light or an electrical charge. The energy causes the oxygen molecules to split, but they rapidly reassemble into a gas that contains both oxygen (O_2) and ozone (O_3). This mixture is used in ozone therapy.

How Does Ozone Therapy Work?

Ozone therapy works on a simple idea: once it enters the body, usually through an intravenous (IV) line (called autohemotherapy), it reacts with molecules in the body and forms substances called ozonides. Ozonides can penetrate cell membranes and speed up certain reactions. Overall, ozone therapy has many benefits for people who have autoimmunity, as well as those who have cancer, infectious disease, and a suppressed immune system. It:

- Stimulates the production of white blood cells, which fight infections
- Enhances the efficiency of antioxidant enzymes, which help rid the body of free radicals
- Fights viruses
- Helps increase the amount of oxygen delivered from the blood to cells, which promotes healing and relieves fatigue
- Helps stimulate basic metabolism, which improves energy levels
- Increases the production of interferon and tumor necrosis factor, which the body uses to fight infections and cancer

- Reduces inflammation
- Oxidizes toxins and thus may aid in their being eliminated from the body
- Normalizes (modulates) production of hormones and enzymes

Ozone therapy combines well with chelation and biodetoxification, and I include it as part of a patient's treatment program at the Edelson Center when appropriate.

What's It Like to Get Ozone Therapy?

At the Edelson Center, I administer autohemotherapy. The IV takes about thirty minutes and involves mixing a measured amount of ozone gas with 100 to 300 cc of the person's blood, and then infusing the ozone/blood mixture into the bloodstream. Some people experience some temporary tightness in their shoulder or chest or have a cough during treatment. Others experience no discomfort.

Treatment may be daily for a month, then weekly, then monthly, depending on the person's illness and response. Symptoms such as nausea, headache, and muscle aches are common and may last for weeks or even months, depending on how toxic the individual is. These symptoms are "healing effects," and are a clear indication that the body is healing from the therapy's many effects. A high dose of vitamin C one hour after treatment helps further suppress free-radical activity, but it is an expensive option.

❖ INTRAVENOUS GAMMA GLOBULIN

If you have ever donated blood to a blood bank, there's a chance that antibodies called immunoglobulins, produced by B-cells in your immune system, were isolated from your donation. They were then purified and mixed with the antibodies from dozens of other donors to create a homogenized pool of antibodies referred to as gamma globulin.

Gamma globulin has been used as a form of therapy since 1952. It has proved effective in the treatment of various auto-immune disorders, including rheumatoid arthritis, lupus, multiple sclerosis (and various other demyelinating conditions such as chronic inflammatory demyelinating polyneuropathy), Kawasaki disease, myasthenia gravis, and autism, yet scientists have not identified exactly how gamma globulin works in the treatment of autoimmunity.

Using Intravenous Gamma Globulin

When used to treat autoimmune conditions, gamma globulin is injected directly into the bloodstream, where it mixes with the patient's own blood and antibodies. Researchers theorize that gamma globulin may have an anti-inflammatory effect, that it neutralizes cytokines (which means it may help stop abnormal immune cell activity), or that it may suppress the production of various autoantibodies, as well as a few other benefits for people with autoimmunity. In animal studies, IV gamma globulin promotes remyelination of nerves in diseases like multiple sclerosis and chronic inflammatory demyelinating polyneuropathy.

The chosen dosage varies and depends on the needs and tolerance of each individual patient. Typically we gradually build up to a maintenance dose and make adjustments as needed. Patients are usually treated for at least six months.

Side effects occur in no more than 10 percent of people who undergo gamma globulin treatment, and may include aseptic meningitis, nausea, vomiting, dizziness, or tachycardia (rapid heartbeat). Severe allergic reactions are extremely rare (less than

0.1 percent), as is the risk of stroke or pulmonary embolism. Gamma globulin can also trigger a migraine attack in people with a history of the condition.

Gamma globulin therapy is considered investigational (for most conditions) in the United States, thus this very expensive treatment program (about $100–$150 per gram, which includes all materials and nursing care) may not be covered by your insurance company.

Gamma Globulin and Autism

Although I wish I could say that intravenous gamma globulin can help every child who has autism, research does not support that idea. So far, studies suggest that it can result in a significant improvement in a small number of autistic children, and that there is a better chance of success if treatment is started early in the course of the condition. It may only improve the abnormal molecular characteristics of the condition and not help with the symptoms.

❖ HUMAN GROWTH HORMONE

Human growth hormone (HGH) is one of the many hormones, like estrogen, progesterone, melatonin, and DHEA, whose level in the body declines with age. HGH is the most abundant hormone secreted by the pituitary gland, which lies deep within the brain. Peak production is during adolescence, when we tend to grow the most, and then it steadily diminishes. By the time we reach age sixty, for example, we secrete about 25 percent of the HGH secreted at age twenty. Thus, in an effort to fight the negative effects of aging, some people take growth hormone supplements to raise the levels of HGH in their body.

How Natural HGH Works in the Body

Natural growth hormone is released into the body in spurts that occur during the beginning phases of sleep and after exercise. Once the pituitary gland releases the hormone, the liver quickly (after a few minutes) converts much of it into a metabolite called insulin-like growth factor type 1 (IGF1). Thus, HGH itself does not exist for very long in the body, and it is actually IGF1 that provides the beneficial effects. In addition, because HGH levels in the body are extremely difficult to measure because of its short life, IGF1 levels are identified to help us know how much HGH the body is producing, as it remains in the bloodstream for twenty-four to thirty-six hours.

Although normal adult levels of IGF1 range from 200 to 450 ng/ml (nanograms per milliliter of blood), many people have even lower levels, including individuals with autoimmune disorders. Abnormally low levels of IGF1 are associated with fatigue, loss of muscle and bone strength, reduced healing capacity, diminished memory and cognitive function, weight gain, and loss of skin tone.

Treatment with HGH

At the Edelson Center, we use HGH when individuals are tested and show abnormally low levels of the hormone for their age. Often, such low levels are seen in people who have lupus or chronic fatigue and immunodeficiency syndrome. HGH is given via injection and should only be used under medical supervision. It can provide a variety of benefits, including the following (not everyone experiences all these effects):

- Improves wound healing
- Reduces fatigue

- Stimulates bone formation
- Increases resistance to infection
- Improves skin tension, thickness, and elasticity
- Reduces facial wrinkles
- Increases lean body mass (reduces fat tissue)
- Improves sex drive
- Improves energy level and exercise performance
- Stimulates organ growth
- Improves sleep
- Enhances mood
- Increases memory retention

Prescription HGH, which is made in a laboratory using a method called recombinant DNA technology, is injectable. This is the form used at the Edelson Center and by clinical molecular physicians who include it as part of their treatment for certain autoimmune patients. There are also HGH enhancers available over the counter. These products work by supplying the body with substances known to increase the body's natural production of HGH. Even though they are available over the counter, they should never be taken without the knowledge of your physician.

❖ CHINESE HERBS

The tradition of Chinese herbal medicine has withstood the test of time for more than four thousand years. Although ancient and even more modern people and scientists didn't understand exactly how or why certain herbs had healing abilities, the apparent fact that they did was enough for them. Today, we have the technology to test the herbs that have been the pillar of medicine in Asia for millennia and that are now being used increasingly throughout the world.

Some Chinese herbs have become household words and can be found in most health food stores and pharmacies, and are being recommended and dispensed by various healthcare professionals. Here are a few that have been shown to have some immune modulation abilities, as well as other qualities that can be beneficial for people who have autoimmune disorders.

• Astragalus root. In traditional Chinese medicine, astragalus root is used to fight viral infections. It also appears to be helpful in people whose immune systems have been damaged by chemicals or radiation, which makes it an option for people who have chemical toxicity. The best form to take is the dry extract, standardized to contain 0.5 percent 4-hydroxy-3-methoxy isoflavone.

• Dong quai. This herb is regarded as the most important female tonic remedy in Chinese medicine. It can improve energy levels, help resist disease, promote blood circulation, protect the liver against toxins, and stimulate liver metabolism, which enhances detoxification.

• Ginseng. Chinese or Korean ginseng (*Panax ginseng*) contains substances called ginsenosides, which can help relieve fatigue, weakness, and low resistance. People who take ginseng also report improved mental acuity. It may cause insomnia if taken before bedtime.

• Ligustrum (privet) fruit (*Ligustrum lucidum*). Chinese medicine doctors often combine this herb with astragalus root for people who have chronic fatigue or weakness. But it is also taken alone as an excellent digestive aid, which makes it a good treatment for Crohn's disease, ulcerative colitis, or other chronic bowel complaints. Ligustrum also aids liver function.

❖ SOME CLOSING WORDS ABOUT IMMUNOTHERAPY

My experience with the therapies discussed in this chapter is that they have proven effective for treatment of autoimmunity. Before I make the decision to use any one or more of these approaches for a patient, I complete a careful and comprehensive evaluation to determine the proper treatment, dose, and length of treatment. Therefore, no one should take it upon him- or herself to self-treat with any of these therapies, even though some of them are available over the counter. You are encouraged to discuss the possibility of using immunotherapy with a qualified clinical molecular physician.

Closing Comments

❖

In the introduction to this book, I said that perhaps the most important question my patients with an autoimmune condition would ask was: Is there anything I can do to get better? That question haunted me for years. And when I found answers to that question, I knew it was time to share them with everyone who suffers with an autoimmune disease.

Having an autoimmune condition can be a lonely and frustrating experience, a fact I have witnessed and heard time and time again from the hundreds of individuals who have come to me looking for answers. And I want to thank each and every one of them—and you—for allowing me to help, and for helping me better understand the link between autoimmunity and environmental toxins.

It may sound strange for me to be thanking my patients, but the truth is, all of them—and you, too, if you have an autoimmune condition—are part of a new frontier in medicine. That frontier involves exploration of the link between autoimmunity and environmental toxins. It is a new, exciting, and, unfortunately for those who have an autoimmune disease, painful experience. My hope is that this book has made it less painful and offered hope and a new realm of treatment options to all who suffer with an autoimmune condition.

The number of treatment options presented in this book may look daunting, but my hope is that you will view them rather as a wealth of possible ways to heal. Autoimmunity is a complex process, regardless of the disease you are experiencing. And complex conditions require a comprehensive healing approach. My intention was to offer you a wide range of healing options—those you can do on your own, as well as those that require the administration and guidance of a knowledgeable professional. In order for treatment of autoimmunity to be successful, a professionally guided treatment course that includes elimination of heavy metals and other toxins, nutritional support, and immunotherapy is crucial. That course of treatment must be administered by a doctor who understands the link between autoimmunity and environmental toxins and the treatments that can break it.

What is sometimes frustrating for me is that so few doctors have come to recognize this relationship. In a way their reluctance to embrace this concept is understandable: as this book has shown, uncovering an autoimmune process and then treating it can take a long time and requires patience on the part of both the doctor and the patient. It also requires that a physician be willing to become well versed in the areas encompassed in clinical molecular medicine. That requires a lot of work on the part of a doctor. But it's work well worth pursuing when you know that in the end, people who have been misdiagnosed, mistreated, and misunderstood will finally get the help they need and deserve.

The good news is that more doctors and researchers are awakening to the truth about the relationship between our poisoned environment and our health. My hope is that you will take what you have read here and apply what you can on your own, and also find a knowledgeable professional to help you on the rest of your healing journey in this new frontier. If you have any questions about autoimmunity or our treatment program, or if you need help finding a knowledgeable physician, feel free to contact us at:

The Edelson Center for Environmental and Preventive Medicine, Inc.
3833 Roswell Rd., Ste. 110
Atlanta, GA 30342-4432
404-841-0088; 404-841-6416 (fax)
Web site: www.edelsoncenter.com

Glossary

Amrit kalash An Ayurvedic herbal antioxidant. It consists of more than forty herbs and is rich in vitamins C and E, beta-carotene, bioflavonoids, and riboflavin. It is reportedly one thousand times more effective at destroying free radicals than other antioxidants. While most other antioxidants protect the body against only one type of free radical, amrit kalash is said to be the only known antioxidant that protects against the full spectrum of free radicals.

Antibodies Proteins produced by the immune system that attach to objects (antigens) they identify as foreign to the body.

Antigen A structure that is foreign to the body, such as a virus or fungus. The body usually responds to antigens by producing antibodies.

Autoantibodies Substances produced by the body that attack the body's cells instead of foreign invaders.

Autoimmune disease A disease in which the body's immune system overreacts and attacks and damages a part of the body rather than an invading or foreign substance.

Beta-glucan A substance that activates macrophages (special immune system cells), which kill tumor cells, bacteria, viruses, fungi, and other foreign invaders.

Blood-brain barrier A membrane that controls the movement of substances such as toxins from the bloodstream into the central nervous system (brain).

Calcium d-glucarate A natural substance that inhibits an enzyme called beta-glucuronidase. Beta-glucuronidase harms the body by hindering the elimination of toxins and is associated with an increased risk for various cancers. Thus taking calcium d-glucarate helps the body better eliminate toxic chemicals and reduces cancer risk.

Catalase An antioxidant and enzyme that speeds up the breakdown of hydrogen peroxide to water and oxygen, and thus is essential for the detoxication process.

Cytokines Chemicals secreted by T-cells that play a key role in producing inflammation. Types of cytokines include interferons, interleukins, and transfer factors.

Demyelination The damage caused to myelin by chronic inflammation. Demyelination eventually results in nervous system scars, called plaques, that interrupt communication between nerve cells and the rest of the body.

Detoxication The natural removal of toxic substances by the body. This term usually refers to the natural toxin-elimination process performed by the liver; compare with *detoxification.*

Detoxification A process of removing toxic substances from the body, typically with the help of supplements or methods that assist the body's natural detoxication.

DHEA (dehydroepiandrosterone) A naturally occurring hormone that is produced in and secreted by the adrenal glands.

Essential fatty acid A type of fat that must be provided by the diet. There are two general categories, omega-3 and omega-6, and all the types in each category are precursors of prostaglandins.

Eubiotic A state of balance between bad and good bacteria in the gut.

Exophthalmos Bulging eyes, often a symptom of Graves' disease.

Free radical A molecule that has an unpaired electron in its outer orbit. This situation makes the molecule unstable and in constant search for an electron to "steal" to make a pair. Free radicals can cause significant damage to the body's cells, tissues, and organs.

Glutamine An amino acid that helps maintain the integrity of the gastrointestinal mucosal lining and is a major player in phase 2 liver detoxication

Glutathione An antioxidant that is one of the most powerful fighters of oxidative stress. It is critical for overall health and helps protect against damage from pesticides, plastics, benzene, carbon tetrachloride, heavy metals, cigarette smoke, and other toxins.

HEPA (high-efficiency particulate arresting) A type of air filter that can remove nearly 100 percent of pollens, molds, spores, dust, and particulates from the air in a given space.

Human leukocyte antigen (HLA) A "tag" on self-cells—cells that are part of the body—that lets the immune system know that the self-cells belong to the body and that they should not be attacked as foreign or invader cells.

Hypercoagulable state "Hypercoagulable" means thickened blood, which is the result of an abnormal amount of fibrin, a healing substance produced by the body, being deposited in the walls of small blood vessels.

Hyperthyroidism A condition characterized by overproduction of thyroid hormones.

Hypothyroidism A condition characterized by underproduction of thyroid hormones.

Immunoglobulin A type of antibody produced by B-lymphocytes.

Interferon A type of cytokine. There are several kinds, including gamma interferon, which is produced by the immune system and causes worsening of symptoms of multiple sclerosis (MS); and alpha and beta interferons, which appear to suppress the immune system and may be useful in the treatment of MS.

Lipoic acid An antioxidant that can deactivate both fat- and water-soluble free radicals, which no other antioxidant can do. Lipoic acid can also raise levels of glutathione.

Lymph nodes Glandlike structures located throughout the body that help remove foreign substances from the body's tissues.

Lymphocyte A category of white blood cell that performs many functions in the immune system. Some of the major types of lymphocytes include B-lymphocytes, T-lymphocytes, natural killer cells, and macrophages.

Macrophage A type of lymphocyte that performs many functions, including consuming invading organisms and tumor cells, and producing cytokines.

Magnetic resonance imaging (MRI) A noninvasive scanning technique that allows physicians to clearly see brain tissue and the flow of cerebrospinal fluid.

Malabsorption An alteration in the ability of the intestinal tract to absorb nutrients into the bloodstream.

Methyl-cobalamine This form of vitamin B_{12} is essential for protein synthesis and nerve cell health.

Mitochondria A structure in cells that is responsible for energy production.

Molecular mimicry A condition where part of a molecule of a protein closely resembles (mimics) a part of another completely different protein. Thus, if the body is attacking foreign organisms, and there are molecules mimicking those organisms, the body will attack both the bad invaders and what it perceives to be bad invaders.

Myelin A fatty covering that protects nerve cell fibers in the brain and spinal cord. The myelin assists the transmission of chemical messages between the central nervous system and the rest of the body. In multiple sclerosis, myelin is damaged, resulting in blocked or distorted signals.

Myelin basic protein (MBP) This substance is a major component of myelin. One sign of multiple sclerosis is an abnormally high level of MBP in the cerebrospinal fluid, because it is released when myelin breaks down in this disease.

Myelin oligodendrocytes Myelin is produced by nervous system cells called oligodendrocytes, thus autoantibodies against these cells further myelin damage.

N-acetylcysteine A precursor to glutathione and a substance that is especially important during phase 1 liver detoxication.

Naringinine A potent antioxidant that is extracted from citrus and available in supplement form.

Natural killer cell A type of lymphocyte that destroys invading organisms and also produces cytokines.

Oligodendrocytes Cells that make and maintain myelin.

Oxidation The name for the damage done to the body by free radicals.

PCR (polymerase chain reaction) A procedure that rapidly produces copies of DNA for identification purposes. It is used to identify various microorganisms.

Phosphatidylcholine A natural substance that is needed for efficient mental functioning and fat metabolism.

Precursor Something that precedes another.

Probiotics Beneficial bacteria, available in supplement form, taken to restore or maintain healthy flora in the intestinal tract.

Receptor A protein on a cell's surface that allows the cell to identify antigens.

Reverse-osmosis carbon filter A type of water filter that is effective at removing nearly 100 percent of contaminants.

SAM-e (S-adenosylmethionine) A natural substance found in the body that is synthesized from the amino acid methionine. It is involved in many processes, including making cartilage, detoxifying blood, and producing proteins.

Synovium The tissue that lines joint capsules. It produces synovial fluid.

T-cell A type of lymphocyte (immune system cell) that is produced in the thymus gland.

Thymus The master gland, located just above the heart, that is responsible for immune system functioning.

Appendix

Where to Buy Health- and Environmentally Friendly Products

This list is representative of the scores of companies that provide health- and environmentally friendly products. You can search the Internet using key words such as "organic," "natural," and "environmentally friendly" along with the specific type of product you wish to find (e.g., "food," "clothing," "supplements"), for additional resources.

A+ Allergy Supply
8325 Regis Way, Los Angeles, CA 90041
800-86-ALLER
Air-purifying products, pet care products, vacuum cleaners, water purifiers

Allergy Alternative
440 Godfrey Dr., Windsor, CA 95492-8036
800-838-1514

Air-purifying products, personal hygiene, supplements, water purifiers

The Allergy Store
PO Box 2555, Sebastopol, CA 95473
707-832-6202
Air filters and purifiers, bedding, childcare products, cleaning products, health and beauty, supplements, building materials, makeup, personal hygiene, supplements, water purifiers

AllerMed
31 Steel Rd., Wylie, TX 75098
214-442-4898
Air-purifying products

American Environmental Health Foundation Inc.
8345 Walnut Hill Ln. #200, Dallas, TX 75231
800-428-aehf
www.aehf.com
Bedding, building materials, cleaning products, clothing, housewares, nontoxic art supplies, personal hygiene, pet care products, footwear, supplements, water purifiers

Aubrey Organics
4419 N. Manhattan Ave., Tampa, FL 33614
800-282-7394
Personal hygiene

Biological Control of Weeds
1140 Cherry Dr., Bozeman, MT 59715
406-586-5111
Pesticide alternatives

The Body Shop
45 Horsehill Rd., Cedar Knolls, NJ 07927-2003
800-541-2535
Personal hygiene

Care2
www.care2.com/shopping
Source of natural household products, bedding, pest control, health and beauty items, furniture, filters

The Company Store
500 Company Store Rd., La Crosse, WI 54601
800-323-8000
Bedding, childcare products, clothing

Eco Directory
www.naturalfoodsdirectory.com
Lists dozens of sources of organic foods, cruelty-free products, herbs, household products, and eco-travel

EcoSource
PO Box 1656, Sebastopol, CA 95473
800-274-7040
Air-purifying products, bedding, building materials, cleaning products, makeup, personal hygiene, pesticide alternatives, supplements, water purifiers

Ecology Box
2260 S. Main St., Ann Arbor, MI 48103
800-735-1371
Bedding, building materials, cleaning products, personal hygiene

Greenpeople Directory
www.greenpeople.org/healthfood.htm
Listings of food co-ops, health food stores, and natural food stores in the U.S.

Heart of Vermont
The Old Schoolhouse
Route 132, Box 183, Sharon, VT 05065
800-630-4123
Bedding, cleaning products, clothing, furniture, housewares, rugs and carpets, footwear

Heavenly Heat
272 Neptune Ave., Encinitas, CA 92024
800-533-0523
Saunas

Janice Corporation
198 Route 46, Budd Lake, NJ 07828
800-526-4237
Bedding, clothing, footwear, housewares, personal hygiene, rugs and carpets

Karen's Nontoxic Products
1839 Dr. Jack Rd., Conowingo, MD 21918
800-527-3674
Bedding, building materials, childcare products, cleaning products, makeup, personal hygiene, pesticide alternatives, supplements

Living Source
7005 Woodway Dr. #214, Waco, TX 76712

817-776-4878
Air-purifying products, bedding, childcare products, cleaning products, clothing, organic food, heating and cooling systems, housewares, makeup, personal hygiene, pesticide alternatives, supplements, water purifiers

N.E.E.D.S.
527 Charles Ave., Syracuse, NY 13209
800-534-1380
Air-purifying products, supplements, water purifiers

Nontoxic Environments
9392 S. Gribble Rd., Canby, OR 97103
503-266-5244
Air-purifying products, bedding, building materials, heating and cooling systems, housewares, personal hygiene, rugs and carpets, supplements

Nordic Naturals
800-662-2544
www.nordicnaturals.com
Toxin-free fish oil capsules

Organic Way Market
120 Peter Lyall, Williamsburg, VA 23185
757-229-2665; 757-258-5412 (fax)
www.theorganicwaymarket.com
Organic food, clothing, baby toys, supplements, furniture, pet products

Priorities
70 Walnut St., Wellesley, MA 02181

800-553-5398
Cleaning products, vacuum cleaners

Real Goods
Ukiah, CA 95482-5507
800-762-7325
www.realgoods.com/index.cfm
Air-purifying products, bedding, solar systems, makeup, personal hygiene, rugs and carpets

Safer Alternatives
19675 Day Ln., Redding, CA 96003
916-243-1352
Air-purifying products, bedding, building materials

Seventh Generation
Colchester, VT 05446-1672
800-456-1177
Automobile products, bedding, building materials, childcare products, cleaning products, paper products, personal hygiene, rugs and carpets

Wellness, Health & Pharmaceuticals
2800 S. 18th St., Birmingham, AL 35209
800-227-2627
Bedding, cleaning products, makeup, personal hygiene, supplements

Organic Foods

Ecology Sound Farms
42126 Road 168, Orosi, CA 93647
209-528-3816

The Green Earth
2545 Prairie, Evanston, IL 60201
800-332-3662

Harbor House Organic Coffee
800-541-4699

Organic Food Shopper
1578 W. Lewis, Dept. E, San Diego, CA 92103
619-425-2813

Organic Wholesaler's Directory & Yearbook
Box 464, Davis, CA 95617

Oshwa American Macrobiotic Foods
PO Box 3608, Chico, CA 95927
916-342-6050

Sunrise Health Food Store
17650 Torrance, Lansing, IL 60438
708-474-6166

Resources for Information on Environmental Toxins

American Academy of Biological Dentistry
408-659-5385

Chemical Injury Information Network
PO Box 301, White Sulphur Springs, MT 59645
406-547-2255
www.ciin.org

Chemical Manipulation of Consciousness, Behavior, Health, and
Evolutionary Potential in the Human Population
See www.trufax.org/menu/chem.html
Many links on this site

Environmental Dental Association
800-388-8124

Environmental Health Clearinghouse
800-643-4794

Environmental Research Foundation
PO Box 5036, Annapolis, MD 21403
Fax: 415-263-8944
e-mail: erf@rachel.org

The Healthy House Institute
www hhinst.com/index.html

International Academy of Oral Medicine and Toxicology
407-298-2450

National Coalition Against the Misuse of Pesticides
701 E St. SE #200, Washington, DC 20003
202-543-5450
www.beyondpesticides.org

Pesticide Hotline
800-858-7378

Preventive Dental Health Association
http://emporium.turnpike.net/P/PDHA/health.htm

Sustainable Alternatives to Pesticides
www.igc.org

Resources for Disease-Related Information

American Autoimmune Related Diseases Association
22100 Gratiot Ave., E. Detroit, MI 48021
800-598-4668
www.aarda.org

American Diabetes Association
1701 N. Beauregard St., Alexandria, VA 22311
800-DIABETES
www.diabetes.org

American Foundation of Thyroid Patients
18534 N. Lyford, Katy, TX 77449
281-855-6608
www.thyroidfoundation.org

Crohn's and Colitis Foundation of America
386 Park Ave. South, 17th Fl., New York, NY 10016
800-932-2423
www.ccfa.org

Lupus Foundation of America
1300 Piccard Dr., Ste. 200, Rockville, MD 20850-4303
800-558-0121
www.lupus.org

Multiple Sclerosis Foundation
6350 N. Andrews Ave., Fort Lauderdale, FL 33309-2130

Helpline: 888-MSFOCUS
www.msfacts.org

Myasthenia Gravis Foundation
5841 Cedar Lake Rd., Ste. 204, Minneapolis, MN 55416
800-541-5454
www.myasthenia.org

National Institute of Diabetes and Digestive and Kidney Diseases
Office of Communications and Public Liaison, NIDDK, NIH,
Building 31, room 9A04
31 Center Dr., MSC 2560, Bethesda, MD 20892-2560
www.niddk.nih.gov

National Multiple Sclerosis Society
733 Third Ave., New York, NY 10017
800-344-4867
www.nationalmssociety.org

National Institute of Arthritis and Musculoskeletal and Skin
Diseases
www.niams.nih.gov/

National Organization for Rare Disorders (NORD)
55 Kenosia Ave., PO Box 1968, Danbury, CT 06813-1968
800-999-6673
www.rarediseases.org

Scleroderma Foundation
12 Kent Way, Ste. 101, Byfield, MA 01922
Info line: 800-722-4673
www.scleroderma.org

Sjögren's Syndrome Foundation
8120 Woodmont Ave., Ste. 530, Bethesda, MD 20814
800-4SJOGREN
www.sjogrens.com

Thyroid Foundation of America
Ruth Sleeper Hall, RSL 350, 40 Parkman St., Boston, MA 02114
800-832-8321
www.tsh.org

Thyroid Society for Education and Research
7515 S. Main St., Ste. 545, Houston, TX 77030
713-799-9909
www.the-thyroid-society.org

Worth Reading

❖

Ashford, N. A., and Miller, C. S. *Chemical Exposures: Low Levels and High Stakes.* New York: Van Nostrand Reinhold, 1998.

Baker, S. M. *Detoxification and Healing: The Key to Optimal Health.* New Canaan, Conn.: Keats, 1998.

Colburn, T., Dumanosky, D., and Myers, J. *Our Stolen Future.* New York: Dutton, 1996.

Edelson, Stephen, M.D. *Living with Environmental Illness.* Dallas: Taylor Publishing, 1998.

Goldberg, Burton, et al. *Chronic Fatigue, Fibromyalgia and Environmental Illness.* Tiburon, Calif.: Future Medicine Publishing, 1998.

Krimsky, S. *Hormonal Chaos: The Scientific and Social Origins of the Environmental Endocrine Hypothesis.* Baltimore: Johns Hopkins University Press, 2000.

Lawson, Lynn. *Staying Well in a Toxic World: Understanding Environmental Illness, Multiple Chemical Sensitivities, Chemical Injuries, and Sick Building Syndrome.* Lynn Lawson, 1994.

———. *Staying Well in a Toxic World: A New Millennium Update.* Lynn Lawson, 2000.

Majamaa, H., and Isolauri, E. "Probiotics: A Novel Approach in the Management of Food Allergy." *Journal of Allergy and Clinical Immunology* 99(1997):179–85.

Moore, Sharon. *Lupus: Alternative Therapies That Work.* Rochester, Vt.: Healing Arts, 2000.

Ohm, Jeanne, D.C., F.I.C.P.A. "Mercury Toxicity in the Unborn and Young." At www.icpa4kids.com/pediatric_chiropractic_articles_mercury_toxicity_in_the_unborn_and_young. htm

Rogers, Sherry, M.D. *Chemical Sensitivity: Environmental Diseases and Pollutants: How They Hurt Us, How to Deal with Them.* New Canaan, Conn.: Keats Publishing, 2000.

———. *Tired or Toxic?* Syracuse, N.Y.: Prestige, 1990.

———. *Wellness Against All Odds.* Syracuse, N.Y.: Prestige, 1994.

Sehnert, Keith W., M.D., et al. "Is Mercury Toxicity an Autoimmune Disorder?" At www.thorne.com/townsend/oct/mercury.html.

Sosin, A., and Jacobs, B. L. *Alpha Lipoic Acid: Nature's Ultimate Antioxidant.* New York: Kensington Books, 1998.

Stoff, Jessie, and Pellegrino, C. R. *Chronic Fatigue Syndrome: The Hidden Epidemic.* New York: Random House, 1998.

Wargo, J. *Our Children's Toxic Legacy: How Science and Law Fail to Protect Us from Pesticides.* Yale University Press, 1996/1998.

Index

Abdominal cramping, bloating, gas, 4, 16, 193, 273
ACTH (adrenocorticotropic hormone), 179
Alcohol, 285
Allergies
    autism and, 65
    avoidance diet for, 95–96, 137–38, 182, 229
    Crohn's disease, ulcerative colitis, and, 155, 160
    enzyme potentiated desensitization (EPD), 301–5
    food, 52, 93, 122, 182, 184
    immunotherapy for, 70
    inhalant, 93
    lupus and, 93, 301–2
    multiple sclerosis and, 182, 184
    testing, 49, 52, 53
Aloe vera, 159
Aluminum, 237
Amino acids, 279
Amrit kalash, 227
Anemia, 81, 95, 158
Ankylosing spondylitis, 186–88
Antibiotics, 154
Antioxidants and antioxidant therapy, 11, 113, 114, 116, 140, 162 , 231, 272, 274–80
    critical, specific antioxidants, 276–79
    dosages, 295–96
    fruits and vegetables, 283
    helpers, 279–80
Apathy, 106
Appetite, 16, 104, 204
Arsenic, 237
Attention span decrease, 104, 106, 214
Autism, 17–18, 59–74
    as autoimmune disorder, 61–62
    case history, 69–70
    causes, triggers, and risk factors, 62–64
    diagnosis and treatment, conventional, 65–68
    evaluation, Edelson, 68–69
    gamma globulin treatment, 312
    as growing epidemic, 59, 60
    signs and symptoms, 64–65
    testing, 39, 50, 55–56, 68–69
    treatment, Edelson, 70–72, 251
    what you can do now, 73–74
Autoimmunity, xi, 9–10, 14, 15
    autoantibodies, 9, 45–47
    autoimmune process, 13–14, 213
    autoimmune response, 9, 12
    causes, xiii, xv, xvi, 4, 10, 42
    conventional treatment, of symptoms, xiii, 10

diagnosis, conventional, xii
factors in, 22–25
number of conditions caused by, 9–10
treatment (three-pronged), 25–26
women and, xi
See also specific disorders

Back pain, 187
Baker's cyst, 124
Balance and coordination, 175
Bauman, Edward, 115
Benzene, 21, 238
Beta-carotene, 276–77
dosage, 295
Beta-glucan, 227
Beta-glucuronidase, 302–3
Biodetoxification, 25–26, 43, 235–65
nutritional therapies and, 268–69
See also Chelation; Colon hydrotherapy;
Environmental controls; Exercise;
Massage; Nutritional therapy; Sauna
Bladder problems, 17, 174
Blood
abnormal clotting, 81
abnormalities and lupus, 85, 90–91
anemia, 81, 158
in stool, 149, 150
vessels, inflammation of (vasculitis),
203–5
Boron, dosage, 296
Bowel, detoxification through, 243

Cadmium, 21, 237
Caffeine, 286
Calcium
d-glucurate, 227, 279
dosage, 296
Cancer
rheumatoid arthritis and, 125
testing, 50
Candidiasis
Crohn's disease and, 158, 159–60
lupus and, 92
multiple sclerosis and, 167
testing, 49, 92
treatment, 229, 306
Catalase, 279
Cat's claw (*uncaria tomentosa*), 272
Chelation therapy, xvii–xviii, 71, 95, 112,

114, 137, 160, 182, 190, 227, 229,
245, 248–52, 254–58
chemicals used in, 250–52
herbal, 97, 115, 140, 161, 184, 230,
254–56
nutritional, 97, 115–16, 140, 161–62,
184, 230–31, 257–58
Chinese herbs, 314–15
Chlamydia pneumoniae, 211–12
Chloroform, 238
Chronic fatigue and immune dysfunction
syndrome (CFIDS), 15–16, 207–31
as autoimmune disease, 210
autoimmune process in, 213–14
causes, triggers, and risk factors, 211–14,
225
conditions that share symptoms with,
220
contagion by, 210–11
course of the disease, 216–17
diagnosis, conventional, 217–20
as environmental disease, 208
evaluation and treatment, Edelson
approach, 223–30, 306
facts about, 209
lifestyle changes, 221–23
symptoms and signs, 15, 50, 93, 214–15
testing, 48, 49, 50, 218–20
treatment, conventional, 220–21
viral connection, 211–12
what you can do now, 230–31
Chronic Fatigue Syndrome (Stoff), 209
Chymotrypsin, 158
Circulatory system, 242
Clinical molecular medicine, xiii, xv, 28–29,
316
finding a physician of, 34–36
Coenzyme Q10, 277–78
dosage, 296
Coffee enemas, 256–57
Cognitive and memory problems, 15, 18,
20, 50, 64, 105, 175, 200, 214, 313
Cold, feelings of, 105, 216
Colon, 148, 149
hydrotherapy, 246, 253–54, 259–60
probiotics for, 273
toxic megacolon, 150
See also Crohn's disease and ulcerative
colitis

Colostrum, 299–300
Conquering Autism (Edelson), 69, 74
Constipation, 16, 17, 65, 105, 174, 215
Copper, 280
  dosage, 296
Corticosteroids, 82, 88–89, 133–34, 160,
  272–73
Crohn's disease and ulcerative colitis, 16,
  141–62
  allergies and, 155, 158, 160
  causes, risk factors, and triggers, 144–46
  chelation therapy, 160, 161–62
  colorectal cancer and, 143
  complications, 149–50
  course of the disease, 143
  DHEA supplements, 161
  diagnosis, conventional, 150–52
  diet and, 146, 155–56, 157, 159, 160
  environmental toxins and, 19, 161
  evaluation, Edelson approach, 156–58
  herbal remedies, 161
  lifestyle changes, 154–56
  mycobactrium (MAP) and, 145–46
  stress and, 24, 156
  surgery and, 156
  symptoms and signs, 4, 10, 16, 148–50
  testing, 46, 55, 151–52, 158
  treatment, conventional, 152–54
  treatment, Edelson approach, 158–60
  what you can do now, 160–62
Cysteine, 258, 279

Dairy (cow milk) products, 145–46, 155,
  286
Davis, Jordan, 240
DDT, 238
Depression
  CFIDS and, 215
  lupus and, 82
  misdiagnosing thyroid conditions and,
    108
  multiple sclerosis and, 172
  thyroid conditions and, 104
DHEA, 97, 161, 307–8
Diabetes (type 1, IDDM), 16, 47, 190–92
Diagnosis (evaluation), 27–56
  conventional, xii
  getting to know you, 29–31
  questionnaire, xviii, 31–34

sign or symptom, 30–31
  testing, 36–56
  See also Tests
Diarrhea, 4, 16, 65, 104, 148, 174, 215,
  273
Dicholorobenzene, 238
Diet
  autism, 73
  autoimmune (and good all-around) diet,
    280–81
  autoimmunity and, 23–24
  carbohydrates, 282
  Crohn's disease, ulcerative colitis and,
    146, 155–56, 157, 159, 160
  essential fatty acids (EFAs), 140, 184,
    227, 289–94
  fats, 282–83
  fiber, 283–84, 287
  food additives, 286
  food sources of essential nutrients, 288–89
  foods to avoid, 285–87
  fruits and vegetables, 283
  guidelines for detoxification and health,
    281–89
  immune-damaging substances in, 24
  legumes, 284
  lupus, 95–96, 97
  multiple sclerosis and, 182, 184
  organic, 281, 282, 283, 287
  pancreatic enzymes, 294–95
  protein, 282
  rheumatoid arthritis and, 122
  serving size, 289
  soy foods, 284
  Standard American Diet, 23–24
  thyroid disorders, 113–14
  toxins in, 23–24
  whole grains and cereals, 284–85
Digestive problems, 50
Dizziness, 15, 215, 237
DMARDs, 129, 131–32
DMSO, 138–39

Edelson Center for Environmental and
  Preventive Medicine, xii, xiv, xv, 35,
  37, 69, 201
  autohemotherapy, 310
  biodetoxification program, 236, 244–65
  contact information, 319

Edelson Center for Environmental and
    Preventive Medicine (*cont.*)
  HGH and, 313
  nutritional therapies, 266–67, 269
Emotional instability, 200
Environmental cleanup or controls, 70–71,
    96, 182–83, 226–27, 229, 260–64
Environmental toxins, xiii, xiv–xv, xiv, 10, 19
  arsenic, xiv
  autism and, 62–63
  autoimmune disorders, role in, 18–20
  autoimmune process and, 13–15, 20–21
  CFIDS and, 212
  chemicals (general), xv, 236–37, 238–39
  cigarette smoke, xvi, 91, 122–23
  Crohn's disease and ulcerative colitis, 144–45
  dioxin and PCBs, 102
  epoxy resins, 197
  heavy metals, xv, xvi, 20–22, 169–71,
    186, 236–41
  lupus and, 79–80
  multiple sclerosis and, 168–70
  pesticides, xvi, 19–20, 21, 102, 225
  removing from the body, 25–26
  rheumatoid arthritis, 121–23
  scleroderma and, 197
  thyroid disorders and, 102–3
  toxicity evaluation, 41–42
  workplace exposure, 91
Enzyme potentiated desensitization (EPD),
    301–5
Epstein-Barr virus, 211
Erythropoietin, 95
Essential fatty acids (EFAs), 140, 184, 227,
    289–94
  fish oil, 292, 293–94
  flaxseed oil, 292, 294
  GLA, 293
  oily fish, 293
  rheumatoid arthritis and, 291–92
Exercise, 245, 252–53, 259
Eyes
  bulging, 16, 104, 108
  dry, 203
  inflammation, 187
  puffiness around, 16, 105

Facial expression, dull, 16
Fainting, 216

Fatigue, 4, 15, 16, 17, 20, 50, 81, 104,
    106, 125, 149, 171–72, 189, 191,
    193, 194, 199, 204, 213, 236, 313.
    See also Chronic fatigue and immune
    dysfunction syndrome (CFIDS)
Fever, 15, 16, 17, 81, 125, 187, 204, 216
Fiber, dietary, 283–84, 287
Fistulas, 149
Food additives, 286
Food sources of essential nutrients, 288–89
Formaldehyde, xv, xvi, 21, 238–39
Free radicals, xvii, 11–13
  autoimmune response and, 12
  damage by and autoimmune disorders,
    10, 13
  DNA damage by, 13
  heavy metals and, 21–22
  IBD and, 142–43
  liver function and, 43
  multiple sclerosis and, 168–69
  oxidation, 11, 12–13
  oxidative stress, 11
  rheumatoid arthritis and, 121, 122, 123

Gamma globulin treatment, 71, 94, 183,
    310–12
  autism and, 312
Genetics
  ankylosing spondylitis, 187
  autism, 62–63
  autoimmune hepatitis, 188
  Crohn's disease and ulcerative colitis, 144–46
  heavy metal toxicity and, 22
  lupus, 77–79, 80
  multiple sclerosis, 167
  rheumatoid arthritis, 120–21
  Sjögren's syndrome, 203
  susceptibility to autoimmune disorders
    (general), xiv, xv, 10, 21, 22–23
  thyroid disorders, 101–2
  type of autoimmune disorder and, 22
Ginkgo biloba, 227
Glomerulonephritis, 192–93
  testing, 46, 48
Glucuronate, 43
Glutamine, 160, 271, 280
Glutathione, 43, 227, 257, 278
  level, test, 44
  peroxidase, 280

Glycine, 43
Glycyrrhyzin, 190
Goiter, 104
Graves disease, 16, 39
  diagnosis and treatment, conventional,
    106–10
  evaluation, Edelson approach, 111–12
  iodine and, 102–3
  signs and symptoms, 103–4
  stress and, 103
  testing, 53, 107
  treatment Edelson approach, 112–13
  triggers, 103
  what you can do now, 114–16
Growth hormone, 95, 227
Gulf War illness, 211–12

Hair
  dry, 16
  fine, brittle, 104
  loss, 81, 104, 197, 200
Hashimoto's thyroiditis, 16, 39
  bacteria, *Yersinia enterocolitica* and, 103
  diagnosis, treatment, conventional,
    106–9, 110–11
  evaluation, Edelson approach, 111–12
  signs and symptoms, 105–6
  testing, 53, 107
  treatment Edelson approach, 114
  what you can do now, 114–16
Headache, 193, 204, 214, 236
Hearing problems, 64, 213
Heart
  abnormalities, 81
  enlarged, 16
  failure and arrhythmia, 213
  irregular heartbeat 216, 274
  myocardial problems, 17, 81
  palpitations, 16
  slowed heartbeat, 106
Hepatitis, autoimmune, 188–90
  heavy metals and, 21
  lupus and, 189
  testing, 45, 46, 189
Herpes virus-6, 211
Hexane/heptane/pentanes, 239
Hormones
  lupus, role in, 79–80
  rheumatoid arthritis, role in, 123

Human growth hormone (HGH), 312–14
Human leukocyte antigen (HLA), 13
Hunger, 16, 191
Hypercoagulation, 50
Hypersensitivity, 16, 64
Hypocorticism, 93

Immune system, 3–7, 13
  bone marrow, 5
  cytokines, 7, 8, 48, 142
  HLA, 13
  immunoglubulins (IgG, IgA, IgM, IgD,
    IgE), 7
  interferon, 7
  lymph nodes, 6
  lymphatic system, 6
  lymphocytes (B-cells, T-cells, natural
    killer cells, macrophages), 6–7, 48
  microglia, 8
  skin and mucous membranes, 5
  spleen, 5–6
  suppression and stress, 24
  testing, 45–47, 50
  thymus, 5, 194–95
  unhealthy, symptoms, 4,
  See also Autoimmune disorders
Immunosuppressants, 153–54, 179–80
Immunotherapy, 26, 297–316
  autism, 70
  CFIDS, 229
  Chinese herbs, 314–15
  DHEA, 307–8
  discussing with a physician, 316
  enzyme potentiated desensitization
    (EPD), 301–5
  gamma globulin, intravenous, 310–12
  human growth hormone, 312–14
  ozone therapy, 308–10
  rheumatoid arthritis, 138
  thymus extracts, 305–7
  transfer factor, 298–301
Indigestion, 237
Inflammation
  anti-inflammatory drugs, 152–53
  gamma globulin treatment, 94
  ibuprofen, 114
  in lupus, 85
  testing, 49

Inflammatory bowel disease (IBD), 141–42, 147. *See also* Crohn's disease and ulcerative colitis
Interleukins, 8
Intestinal blocks, 149–50

Joints
    achy (arthralgia), 17, 81, 189
    pain, 17, 124, 187, 200, 204, 214
    stiffness, 17, 124, 187
    swelling, 17
    See also Rheumatoid arthritis

Kanner, Leo, 60
Kidney
    autoimmune diseases of, 46, 48, 192–93
    detoxification and, 244
    lupus and, 46, 47, 81
    testing, 47–48

L-carnitine, 227, 279
Lawrence, Dr. H. Sherwood, 298
Lead, 21, 237
    multiple sclerosis and, 169, 171
Leaky gut syndrome, 26, 269–73
    autoimmune disorders and, 38
    diabetes and, 192
    healing for, 271–72
    probiotics and, 272–73
    rheumatoid arthritis and, 122
    testing for, 37–38
    treatment, 228
    why the gut leaks, 270–71
Lipoic acid, 227, 257–58, 277
Liver
    CFIDS and, 213
    detoxification by, 241–42
    free radical damage and, 43
    nutritional support, 44
    Phase 1, 2 Liver Detoxification Profile, 43–44, 242
    testing, 55
Lumps, 124
Lupus (SLE), 14, 17, 75–97
    African Americans and, 76
    allergies and, 93, 301–2
    as autoimmune disease, 76–77
    causes, triggers, and risk factors, 77–80
    depression and, 82

diagnosis, conventional, 83–87
    evaluation, Edelson, 91–93
    forms of, 77
    heavy metals and, 21
    kidney problems and, 46, 47
    Sjögren's syndrome and, 202
    steroids and, 82, 88–89
    stress and, 24
    symptoms and signs, xvii, 4, 17, 80–83, 84–85, 93
    testing, 45, 46, 47, 49, 86–87, 92–93
    treatment, conventional, 87–91
    treatment, Edelson, 94–97
    what you can do now, 96–97
    women and, 75
Lupus Foundation of America, 75
Lymph nodes, swollen, 15, 214

Magnesium dosage, 296
Malabsorption, 149, 273–74
Malaise, 15, 50, 214
Malnutrition or starvation, 51, 53
Manganese, 280
    dosage, 296
Marth, Jamey, 78
Massage, 246, 253, 259
McEwen, Leonard, 302
Medi-Net, 36
Men
    ankylosing spondylitis in, 186
    polyarteritis nodosa in, 104
Menstruation problems, 104, 216
Mercury toxicity, xvi–xvii, 239–41
    autoimmune diseases associated with, 20, 69–70
    multiple sclerosis and, 169, 171, 182
    signs and symptoms, xvii, 20
    sources of, 20, 69–70, 237
    thyroid conditions and, 112
    vaccinations and, 64, 70
Methyl-cobalamine, 227
Migraine headache, 81
Molybdenum, 280
    dosage, 296
Mouth
    dry, 203
    redness of, 204
    sores, 148
Multiple sclerosis (MS), 17, 163–84

allergies and, 182, 184
as autoimmune disease, 165
causes, triggers, risk factors, 166–70,
171, 182, 211–12
communication, nervous system, and,
164
course of the disease, 165–66
diagnosis, conventional, 175–77
evaluation (Edelson approach), 180–82
gamma globulin treatment, 311
misdiagnosis of, 177
relapsing-remitting phase, 166
signs and symptoms, 17, 170–75
testing, 39, 40, 41, 47–48, 55–56,
176–77, 181–82
treatment, conventional, 178–80
treatment, Edelson approach, 182–83
viral connection, 211–12
vision and urinary problems, 17, 48
women and, 166
Muscle
abnormal movements, 64
aches and pains, 4, 15, 204, 214
atrophy, 274
cramping, 274
foot drop, 170–71
inflammation, 200
weakness, 16, 17, 39–40, 65, 104, 173,
191, 195, 204, 213, 313
Myasthenia gravis, 40, 193–95
testing, 55–56
Mycoplasmas, 121–22, 211–12

N-acetylcysteine, 227, 258, 280
N-acetylglucosamine (NAG), 272
Naringinine, 227
Nausea, 193
Nervous system
lupus and neurological problems, 85
testing for damage, 40
Nervousness, 16
Nickel, xv, 238
Night sweats, 200, 215
NSAIDs, 129, 130–31
Nutritional deficiencies, 93
Nutritional therapies, 70, 94, 113, 137,
246, 258, 266–96
antioxidant therapy, 274–80, 295–96
avoidance diet, 95–96, 137–38, 182, 229

benefits of, 267
biodetoxification and, 268–69
complex, with supplements, 227
foods that suppress thyroid function, 114
inflammatory bowel disease and, 159
leaky gut syndrome and, 269–73
malabsorption and, 273–74
multiple sclerosis and, 183
nutrients, essential, dosages, 296
See also Diet

Oberg, Gary, 169
Obesity, 228–29
Our Stolen Future (Colburn *et al.*), 102
Oxidation, 11, 12–13
P-450 enzymes and, 43
Oxidative stress, 11
profile (test), 44–45
Ozone therapy, 26, 71, 94–95, 137, 160,
190, 246, 308–10

Pain
abdominal, 200
multiple sclerosis and, 172–73, 178–79
Pancreatic enzymes, 71, 96, 294–95
Papanicolaou, Dimitris A., 212–13
Pectin, 160
Phosphatidylcholine, 227
Photosensitivity, 81, 84
Physician, choosing a, 34–36
Pizzorno, Joseph, Jr., 122
Polymyositis, 40, 45, 46, 195–96
Probiotics, 228, 271–73
Progesterone therapy, 227
Proteinuria, 93, 192–93
Public Citizen Health Research Group, 36

Radiation, avoiding, 264
Rash, 17, 77, 81, 84, 150, 204, 216
Raynaud's phenomenon, 81, 196–97
Rectum, 148, 149. *See also* Crohn's disease
and ulcerative colitis
Restlessness, 104
Rheumatoid arthritis, 17, 117–40
autoimmune process and, 119–20
cancer and, 125
causes, risk factors, and triggers, 14,
120–23
course of the disease, 125–26

Rheumatoid arthritis (*cont.*)
  debilitation from, 119, 126
  diagnosis and treatment, conventional,
    126–29
  diseases that mimic, 127
  drug alert, 133
  evaluation, Edelson approach, 134–36
  mycoplasma and, 121–22
  pregnancy and, 39
  silicone immune toxicity syndrome and,
    199
  Sjögren's syndrome and, 202
  symptoms and signs, xviii, 10, 14,
    123–25
  testing, 46, 47, 51, 128, 135–36
  treatment, conventional, 129–34
  treatment, Edelson approach, 136–40
  what you can do now, 140
  women and, 17, 119
Rona, Zoltan P., 38
Rose, Noel R., 25

Salt, 115
SAM-e, 227
Sauna therapy, high temperature
  for autism, 71
  for CFIDS, 227–2
  at Edelson Center, 245, 247
  for Graves' disease, 112
  for Hashimoto's thyroiditis, 114
  home, 258
  for lupus, 95
  for rheumatoid arthritis, 137
Scleroderma, 196–97
  Sjögren's syndrome and, 202
  testing, 45
Seizures, 65, 81, 213, 216
Selenium, 277
  dosage, 296
Sensitivities, 200, 216, 301. *See also*
  Allergies
Serine, 227
Sexual difficulties, 104 , 175
Silicone immune toxicity syndrome,
  197–202
Sjögren's syndrome, 202–3
  silicone immune toxicity syndrome
    and, 199

Skin
  detoxification through, 243
  doscoid lupus and, 77
  dry, 16, 105
  fragility and bruising, 125
  purple spots on, 204
  rash, 17, 77, 81, 84, 150, 204, 216
  thickening, 16, 196
  tone, loss of, 313
Skip lesions, 148
Sleep disorders, 104, 214
Slippery elm (*ulmas fulva*), 272
Sore throat, 15, 214
Spasticity, 173–74, 178
Speech problems, 64, 170, 194
Stamina, lack of, 15
Stiffness, 124
Stress
  autoimmunity and, 24
  CFIDS and, 212–13
  cortisol levels and, 212–13
  Crohn's disease, ulcerative colitis, and,
    156
  Graves' disease and, 103
Stress of Life, The (Selye), 24
Sugar, 285
Superoxide dismutase (SOD), 275, 278–79
Sweating, abnormal, 65
Sweaty palms, 104
Swelling (edema), 105, 197, 274
Systemic sclerosis, 21

Taylor, John-Hermon, 145
Tests, 36–56
  amino acid analysis, 51, 135
  anti-DNA antibody, 45–46, 86, 92
  antineutrophil-cytoplasmic antibody
    (ANCA), 46
  antinuclear antibodies (ANA), 45, 86,
    92, 129, 136, 189
  antiphospholipid antibody (APA), 46–47
  anti-Sm antibody, 46, 86
  anti-smooth muscle antibody (ASMA), 46
  autoimmune thyroid disease, 53–55
  barium enema, 151
  biochemical profile, 51, 92
  blood chemistry, 219
  C-reactive protein (CRP) test, 49, 128,
    136, 151

cardiovascular, pulmonary, genitourinary, 41

CBC (complete blood count), 51, 92, 151, 219

CDSA (comprehensive digestive stool analysis), 37, 92, 135, 151, 158, 224

central nervous system, 39–41

colonoscopy, 151

complement levels, 47, 87

Crohn's disease, 55

cytokine profile (inflammatory), 48

detoxification evaluation, 42–44

DHEA levels, 38, 136

DNA injury, 136

echocardiogram, 92

electroencephlogram (EEG), 40–41

electromyogram (EMG), 39–40

erythocyte sedimentation rate (ESR) test, 49, 128, 151, 219

evoked potentials, 39, 176

gastrointestinal symptoms, 37–38

glomerular basement membrane autoantibody (GBMA), 46

glutathione levels, 44

heavy metal challenge, 41, 92, 135, 158, 224

hemoglobin and hematocrit tests, 128

hormonal system, 38–39

immune complex studies, 47–48

immune studies, 45–47

immune system activation of coagulation test (ISAC), 50

immunoglobulin G radioallergosorbent test (IgG RAST), 52

infectious organism evaluation, 42

islet cell antibodies (ICAs), 47

lactulose mannitol challenge, 37–38, 92

LE cell test, 86–87

lipid peroxide levels, 136

liver, 55

lumbar puncture, 176–77

Lyme serology, 219

MRI (magnetic resonance imaging), 40, 176

natural killer cell activity, 136

nerve conduction velocity, 40

neurological disorders, 55–46

neurotransmitters, 39

nutritional studies, 51–52, 93

organic acid analysis, 51–52

oxidative stress profile, 44–45

Phase 1 and 2 Liver Detoxification Profile, 43–44

rheumatoid factor (RF), 46, 128, 136

sensitivity evaluation, 52–53

sex hormone levels, 38–39

sigmoidoscopy, 151–52

skin testing, 53, 135

T-cell subsets test, 50

TH1-TH2 cytokine profile, 48–49

thyroid blood tests (T4, TSH, anti-TPO), 107, 219

tilt table testing, 219–20

toxic (blood) chemistry studies, 41–42, 92

toxicity evaluation, 41–42, 92, 224

tumor necrosis factor, 136, 142

ulcerative colitis, 44

upper GI series, 151

urinalysis, 92, 219

X-rays, 128

Thirst, excessive, 16, 191

Thymus extracts, 26, 113, 114, 190, 227, 305–7

how they work, 305–6

safety of, 306–7

treatment with, 306

Thyroid, 243

Thyroid conditions, 98–116

as autoimmune disorder, 100–101

causes, triggers, and risk factors, 101–3

diagnosis and treatment, conventional, 106–11

evaluation and treatment Edelson approach, 111–14

Graves' disease, 16, 39, 98–99, 100–101, 102–4

Hashimoto's thyroiditis, 16, 39, 98, 99, 100–101, 103, 105–6

hyperthyroidism, 53, 54, 98

hypothyroidism, 53, 54, 55, 98, 105

misdiagnosing, 108

pregnancy or menopause and, 39

prevalence of, 98

signs and symptoms, 93, 103–6

testing for autoimmune disease, 53–54, 107–8, 112

transient thyroiditis, 99–100

Thyroid conditions (*cont.*)
  what you can do now, 114–16
  women and, 99
Tin, 238
Tingling or numbness (hands, feet), 17, 20,
  165–66, 170, 172, 200, 216
Tinnitus, 216
Toluene, xv, xvi, 239
Toxicology, xv–xvi
Transfer factor, 26, 112–13, 114, 298–301
  colostrum, 299–300
  natural and unnatural, 299–300
  oral, 95
  side effects, 301
  using, 300–301
  who should use, 300
Treatment (Edelson approach)
  antioxidant therapy, xviii, 113, 114, 140,
    162, 184, 272, 274–80
  autism, 70–72
  autoimmune hepatitis, 190
  biodetoxification, 25–26, 43, 235–65
  chelation therapy, xvii–xviii, 71, 95, 112,
    114, 137, 160, 182, 184, 190, 227,
    229, 245, 254–58
  CFIDS, 223–30, 306
  Crohn's disease, ulcerative colitis, IBD,
    158–60
  drug-free, xvii
  immunotherapy, 26, 70, 138, 297–316
  lupus, 94–96
  multiple sclerosis, 182–83
  nutrition and supplement program, 26,
    266–96
  ozone therapy, 308–10
  rheumatoid arthritis, 137–40
  sauna, high temperature, 245, 247
  thyroid disorders, 112–14
  See also specific disorders
Tremors or trembling, 16, 20, 104, 173, 179
Trichloroethylene (TCE), 21, 239

Ulcerative colitis. *See* Crohn's disease and
  ulcerative colitis

Ulcers, 149
Ultraviolet blood irradiation, 227
Urination
  abnormal frequency, infrequency, 16,
    191, 193
  blood in urine, 204

Vaccinations, 64, 72–73
Vasculitis, 46, 47, 93, 203–5
Vision problems, 17, 20, 64, 166, 171,
  174, 194
Vitamin B complex, 279
  dosage, 296
Vitamin C, 277, 310
  dosage, 295
  therapy, 190
Vitamin E, 277
  dosage, 295
Vomiting and cramping, 149, 193

Weight
  gain, 105, 313
  loss, 16, 104, 125, 149, 204, 274
Williamson, Charles, 239, 240
Women
  autoimmune disorders in, xi, 39
  CFIDS in, 209
  giant cell arteritis in, 204
  lupus in, 75
  multiple sclerosis in, 166
  polymyositis in, 195
  pregnancy or menopause, onset of
    autoimmune disease with, 39
  rheumatoid arthritis in, 17, 119
  Sjögren's syndrome in, 202
  thyroid disease and, 99

Xylene, 239

Zinc, 280
  dosage, 296